I0824105

THE WISDOM OF Walking in Nature

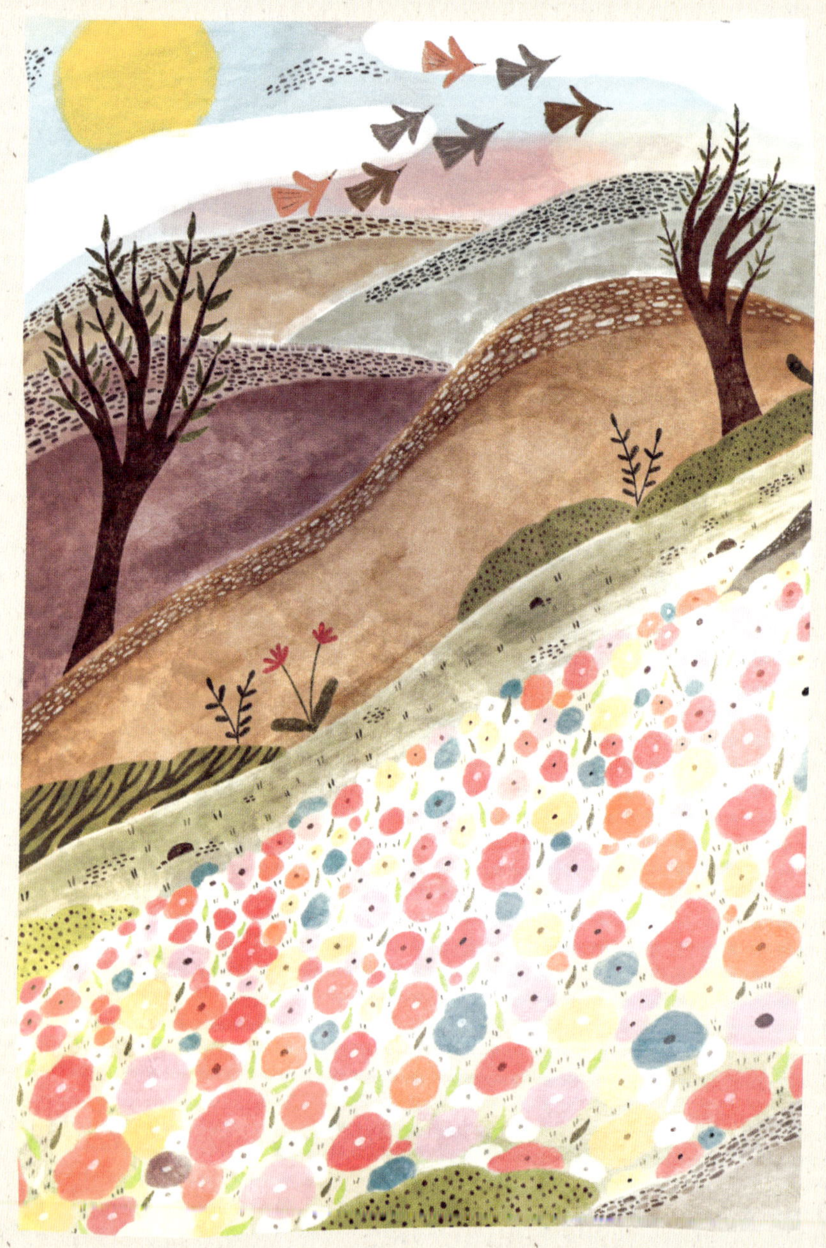

THE WISDOM OF Walking in Nature

50 Mindful & Therapeutic Ways to Enjoy *any* Walk

ALISON DAVIES

ILLUSTRATIONS BY
DOMENIQUE SERFONTEIN

RIZZOLI
UNIVERSE

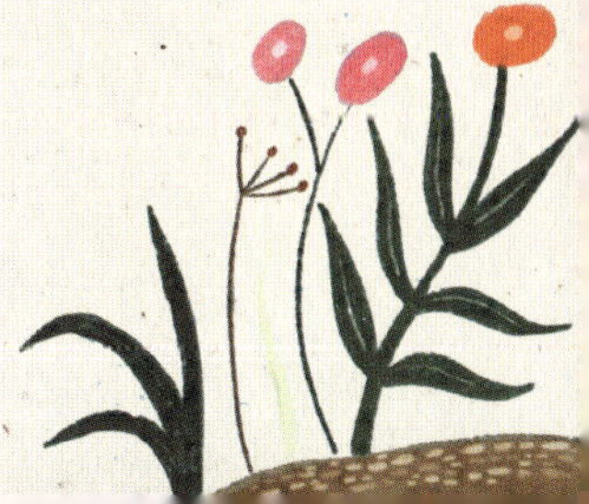

First published in 2026 by
Rizzoli Universe, a division of
Rizzoli International Publications

Rizzoli International Publications Inc
49 West 27th Street
New York, NY 10001

Rizzoli International Publications UK Ltd
Somerset House, West Wing
Strand, London WC2R 1LA

www.rizzoliusa.com

Publisher: Charles Miers
Associate Publisher: Tina Persaud
Senior Editor: Kristy Richardson
Design: Nic + Lou
Production Manager: Michelle Wells

A CIP catalogue record for this book is available from the British Library.

ISBN 978-0-78934-626-1

2026 / 1

Printed in China

The authorized representative in the EU for safety and compliance is Mondadori Libri S.p.A., via Gian Battista Vico 42, Milan, Italy, 20123, www.mondadori.it

Visit us online: Instagram.com/RizzoliBooks
Facebook.com/RizzoliNewYork
Youtube.com/user/RizzoliNY

Contents

CHAPTER THREE: Seaside Walks 74

CHAPTER FOUR: Short Strolls 106

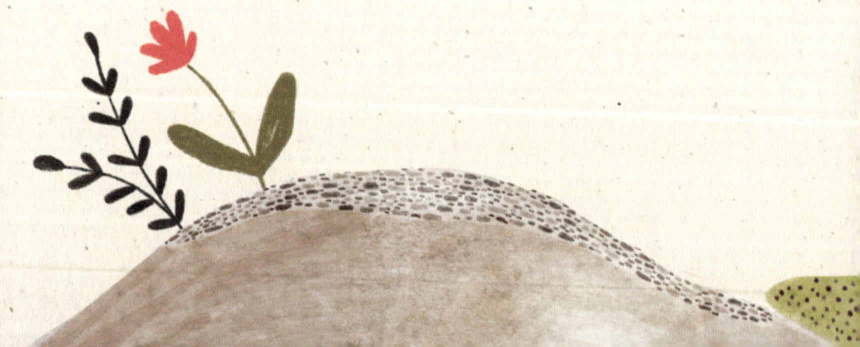

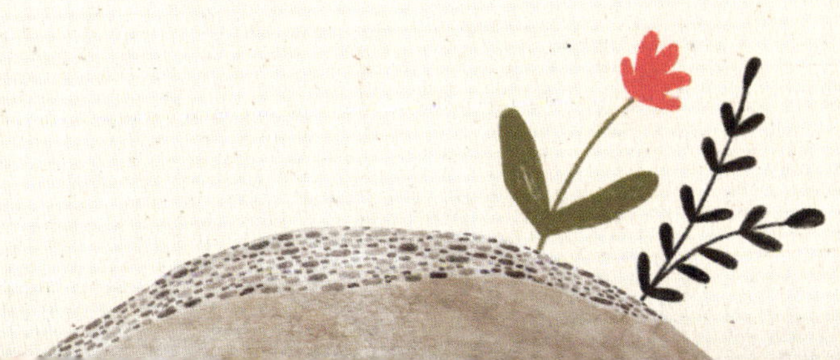

Introduction

Walking is a ritual. It's a way to detach from the chaos of a busy day and an opportunity to be totally present in the moment. It promotes a sense of calm, but it can also be a call to action, a way to invigorate and lighten the mood while fueling the body with vitality. For some, it's a form of exercise; for others, it's a way of life. But although it is a different experience for everybody, depending on the landscape and the walker's aim, there's one thing that remains the same—a walk helps you reconnect with the natural world.

When you take a stroll, you engage with your surroundings at a deeper level. You might not be aware of this at first, but given time to acclimatize you'll begin to notice the little things, such as early morning birdsong peeping between layers of traffic noise as you do your morning commute. You'll enjoy the gentle breeze that strokes your face as you wander through a meadow, or for those more experienced hikers, the undulating, emerald-green hills and golden sunlit valleys on a countryside trek. There is always something new to see and appreciate, and if you're able to make the extra effort, you'll benefit on many levels.

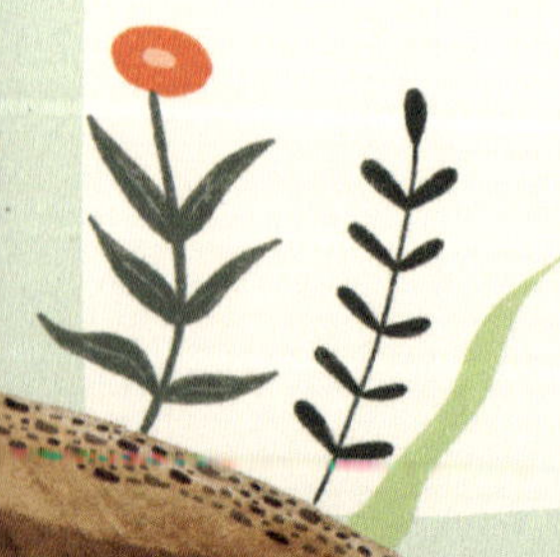

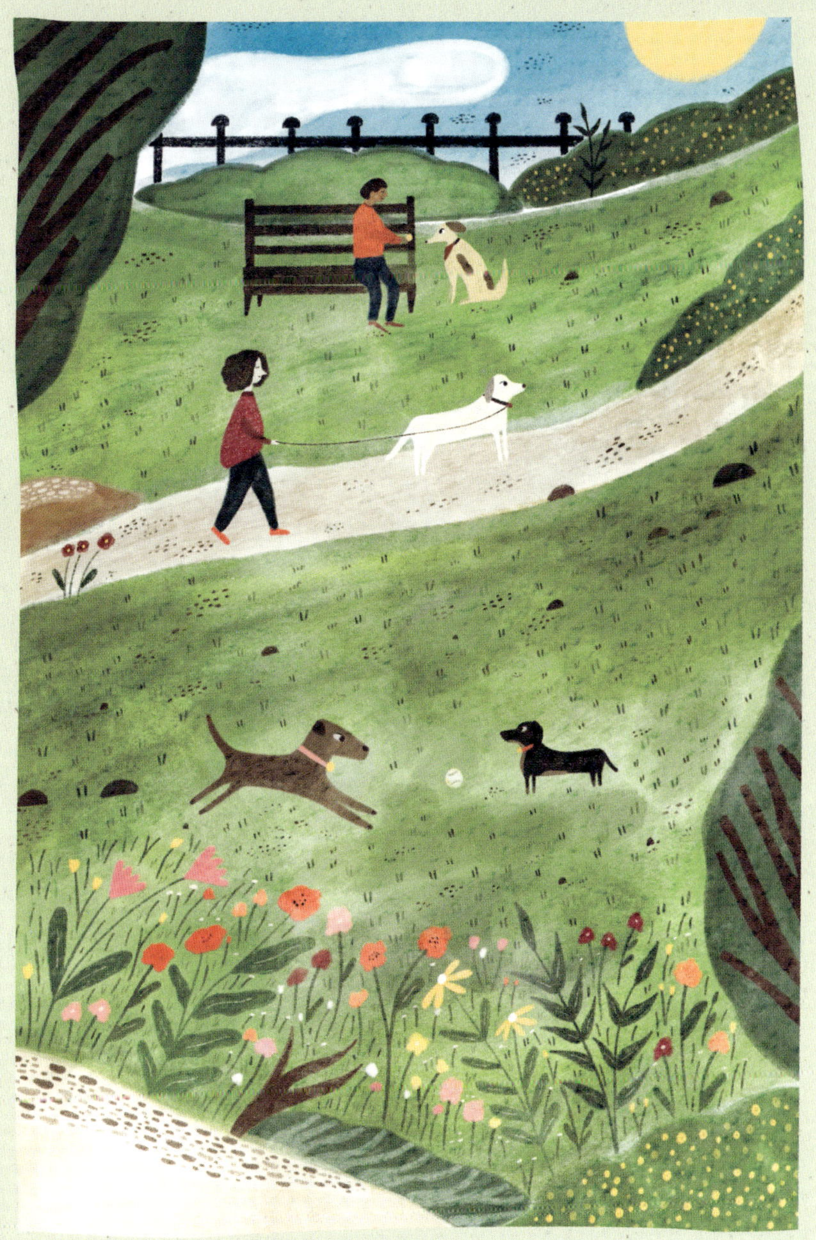

A daily dose of walking, however short, builds inner and outer strength, exercising core muscles and contributing to bone health. The physical activity burns calories and promotes the flow of oxygen and other nutrients around the body. It improves overall circulation and joint mobility, while giving the heart a workout, which in turn lowers blood pressure. It also increases the production of cells that improve the immune system, helping you to fight off infection.

Whether you're pounding the sidewalk in the local park during your lunch hour, or meandering through the woods at the weekend, you'll find that stress hormones dip and feel-good chemicals are released. This mood-boosting combination alleviates anxiety and depression, while promoting relaxation—no wonder sleep patterns improve! But this is only the beginning. If you're prepared to change up your routine and employ mindful and creative techniques when you step out, you'll reap the rewards and discover more about yourself and the environment.

This book explains how you can make the most of any walk. Using the tools at your fingertips to stay present along with engaged and creative techniques that will help you look at things from a fresh perspective, it is arranged into chapters that explore the different types of walks you can enjoy. From woodland rambles, seaside ambles, and urban forays to those longer countryside hikes, waterside walks, and much shorter strolls, the book showcases fifty of the best walks and shows you how to use the time to observe, engage, and reflect in new ways.

It doesn't matter if you're a complete beginner or an advanced hiker, you will learn what to look out for, depending on the landscape, and discover hints and tips to enrich your experience. Practical prompts provide ideas for things you can do before, during, and after your walk. The colorful illustrations that accompany the text will help to inspire and motivate you, and the techniques outlined can be adapted to almost any environment, so you can experiment and see what works for you.

Whether you dip in daily for inspiration or work your way through the walks in each section, there's no set way to read and enjoy this book. Like walking, you dictate the tone and pace. It's entirely up to you where you go and what you do along the way. There is so much wisdom to be found in walking—all you have to do is take that first step.

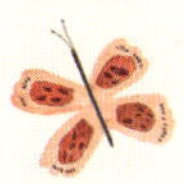

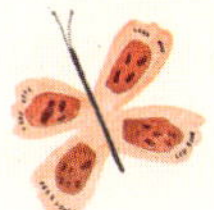

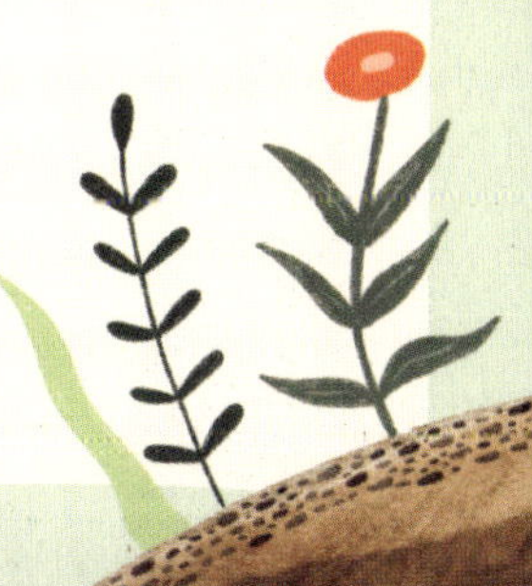

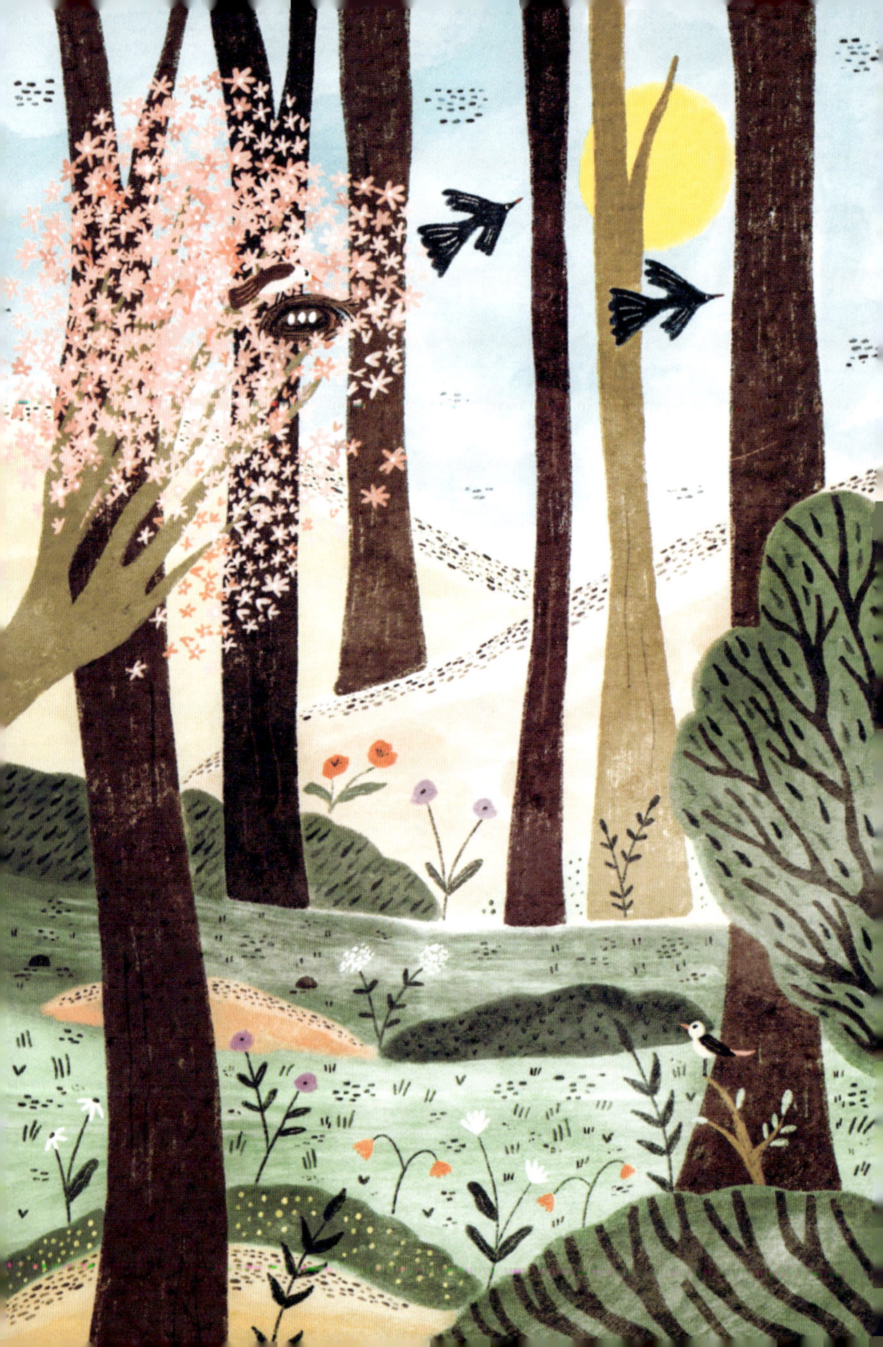

CHAPTER ONE

Woodland Walks

A woodland setting provides a cloak of calm away from the hustle and bustle of everyday life; it is a leafy escape for walkers and offers the perfect backdrop to gather thoughts, clear the head, and trigger the imagination.

Here you'll find an array of mindful suggestions for woodland walks throughout the seasons.

WALK 1

Spring into Spring

A woodland walk is good for you. Being immersed in nature reduces stress and lowers blood pressure. The natural light boosts vitamin D, keeping the immune system in tip-top shape, while also regulating the body clock, which promotes a healthy sleep pattern. A brisk walk increases the heart rate and gets the blood pumping, so your heart will thank you too!

When you walk is just as important as where you take your daily stroll. Evidence suggests a spring amble is deeply therapeutic, thanks to the array of sights, sounds, and smells on offer. Those first stirrings of life, from the unfurling flower buds to the delicate chirp of birdsong, lift the spirits and induce a positive and relaxed mindset.

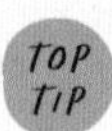

PAUSE FOR THOUGHT

Immerse yourself in the revitalizing energy of spring by taking regular well-being pauses as you walk. Use this time to stand in stillness and feel the peace. Position your feet hip-width apart. Place both hands over your heart in the center of your chest. Draw a long, invigorating breath in through your nose. Imagine you're drinking in the energy of this natural space, letting it permeate your being. Exhale slowly and relax your body.

WALK FOR WELL-BEING

Open your heart and mind and receive the gifts of spring by taking a leisurely stroll through the woods. Treat this as an act of self-care and a way to center yourself. Engage your senses and, most importantly, pay attention to how you feel before, during, and after your walk.

Before you begin, make sure you are wearing the right clothing and footwear. Spring weather can be unpredictable, bringing both sunshine, showers, and chilly winds. Dress in lots of layers, so you will be cozy when it's cold, but you can remove a layer if the sun comes out.

- Take in the general ambience of the woods as you stroll and notice how it makes you feel. Breathe deeply and elongate your spine to stretch out tired muscles.
- Look up at the sunlight filtering through the trees and notice the vibrancy it brings. Look down at the earth beneath your feet and take note of those small changes: how the stony, brittle surface seems to have softened with the extra light and warmth.
- Keep your eyes open for signs of new life. Look out for tiny saplings and new shoots that have emerged from cracks and crevices to greet the sun. See how many buds you can spot and how many flowers have started to bloom. Appreciate their color and beauty, and try to identify them.

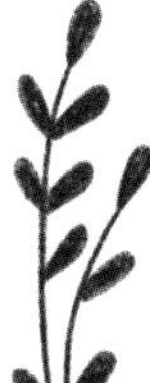

- Make this a complete sensory experience by engaging each of your senses in turn. For example, once you've spotted a flower in bloom and studied its appearance, get closer and see if you can smell its sweet scent. What does it remind you of?
- Take in a deep breath of air: what do you taste on your tongue?
- Close your eyes and listen to the breeze as it blows through the undergrowth. What other sounds can you hear at this time? Know that there is no need to rush, that everything in nature happens at its own pace.
- As you wind your way through the woods, be sure to notice all the changes that come with this new season.

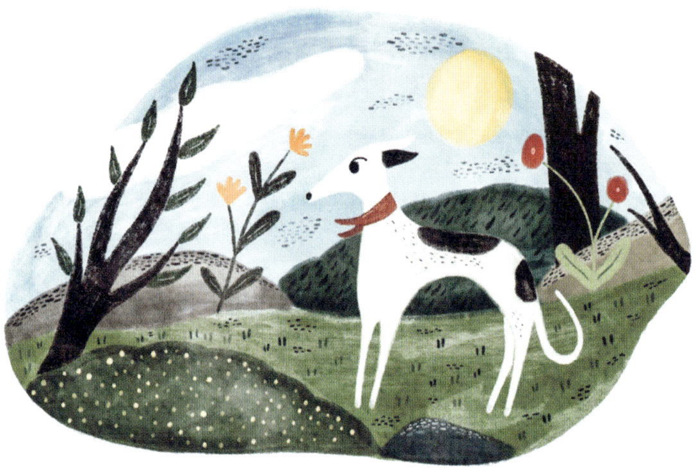

WALK 2

Tell the Trees

Trees have existed since before dinosaurs roamed the Earth. These silent sentinels provide oxygen, store carbon, and regulate the water cycle. They're also a safe haven for wildlife, supporting ecosystems, and providing us with a much-needed retreat from the stresses of daily life. The chemical compounds they release to protect themselves, known as phytoncides, boost the immune system, and help to lower blood pressure and the stress hormone cortisol. No wonder a woodland walk makes you feel so good!

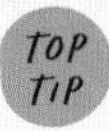

FIND YOUR TREE

Ancient peoples believed that trees were sacred. They thought of them as spiritual guardians with magical properties. The willow, in particular, was thought to be the keeper of secrets and the tree to share your problems with. All trees resonate with a peaceful energy and can help you feel calmer and adopt a more positive mindset.

During your walk, look out for a tree that calls to you personally. Whatever type of tree it is, sit or stand beneath its boughs and look up. Lean your back against the trunk and feel the bark support you. Take a long, deep breath in, and, as you exhale, release any fear or anxiety that you are holding on to. If you feel inclined, tell the tree a secret or a worry that is bothering you, then relax and enjoy spending time with this natural wonder.

THE TREE OF KNOWLEDGE

Enhance your woodland forays by walking among the trees. Observe their mighty presence, while getting to know them a little better. You'll benefit in so many ways. From improving your observation skills, so you can identify your favorites, to understanding their true nature and connecting with them at a deeper level, you'll realize that the trees have all the answers.

- To help you identify each tree, invest in a pocket guide that is easy to carry on your walks. It's a good idea to research the woodland beforehand, so you know what types of trees you're likely to find. Once you have done this, you might choose to set an intention. For example, you might be looking for a specific type of birch or beech, or perhaps you know there's a copse of ancient oaks hidden away at the heart of the wood, and you're hoping to find them. That said, don't let this blind you to the beauty of the other trees on your walk.

- Be open as you walk and focus your gaze on the trees that line the path. Look at the whole tree: notice the root structure, the base of the trunk, and follow this up to the canopy. Take in the size and stature, and let those first impressions come. How does the tree make you feel?

- Take note of the tree's bark. Look at its color, and reach out and run your hand over it to find out if it is rough or smooth. Some trees are hardier than others, depending on where they grow. Also check out the leaves, looking at how they are formed, as well as their size and shape. Notice the color and seek out any distinguishing marks.

- Depending on the time of year, the tree may be in fruit, so use these as clues to the type of tree you have found. Make a note of your discoveries, so you can look them up in more detail when you get home.

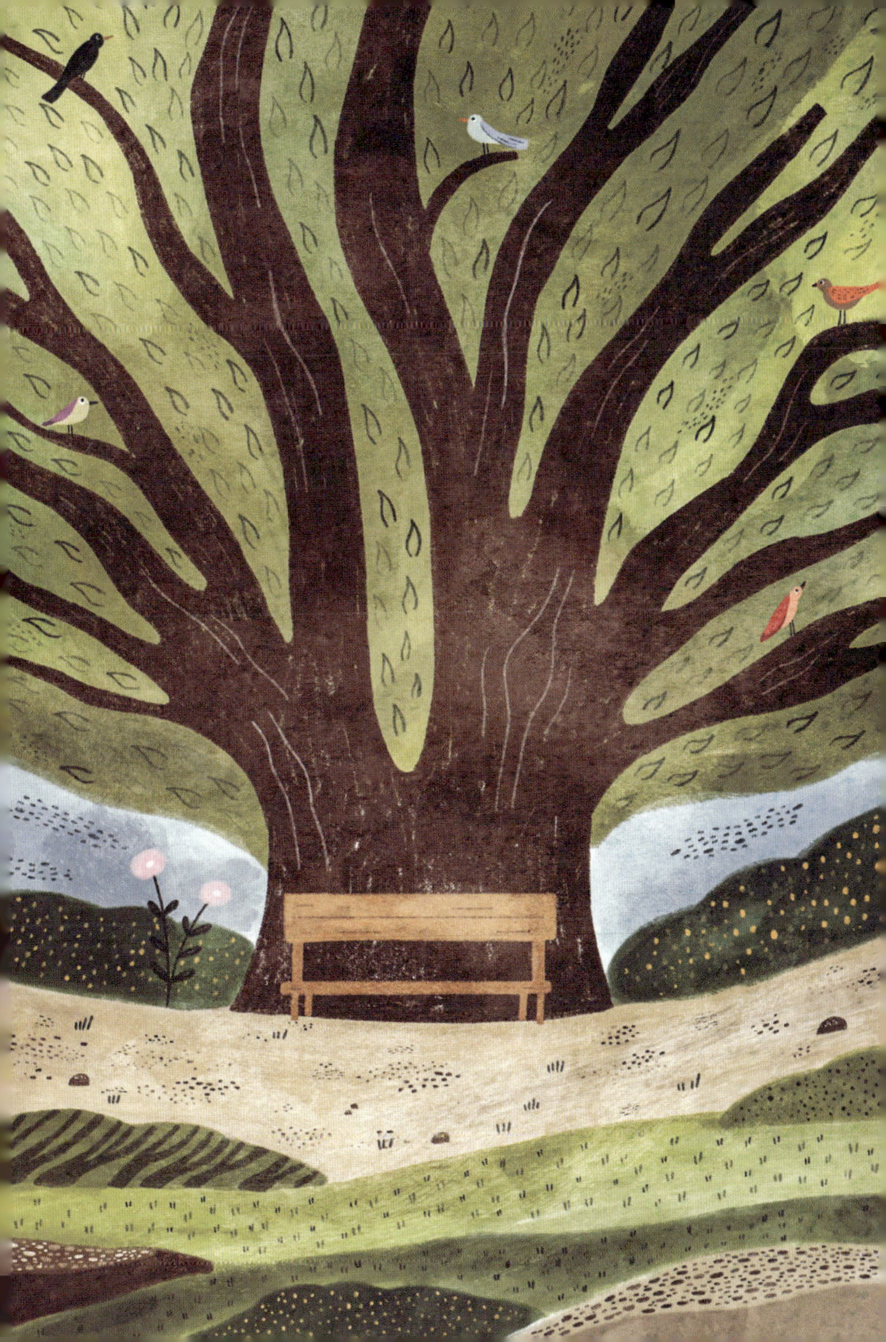

WALK 3

Autumn Ramble

Autumn is the seasonal shapeshifter. It sweeps through the landscape, bringing a rich and vibrant carpet of colors. Jewel tones abound, as the lush, zingy greens of summer are swapped for a palette of burned orange and deep mauve tones. The air is heavy with moisture and feels much cooler against the skin. It is time to pull out the winter woollies, don hardy walking boots, and wear thick, fleecy scarves. The ground is brittle as the soil hardens against the elements. The trees are shedding their leaves in readiness for the chill of winter.

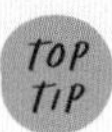

RECORD YOUR MEMORIES

In this walk you are making memories, recording each feature by focusing on it and tagging it with a descriptive sentence. Take this a step further by finding a memento for everything that you notice. For example, if you love the vibrant leaves, you might pick one that stands out in color and shape and take it home with you. If you can hear the snap of twigs at your feet, you might find a small one to carry. A fallen feather might remind you of the feeling of the wind brushing gently against your skin. If you can smell the earth, dig down and find a stone to help you make that connection with the mud and soil.

SENSORY STROLL

Despite the changes in weather, autumn is one of the most popular times of the year to take a woodland walk. The seasonal transition is a sensory delight. It provides an opportunity to explore and get up close and personal with the natural world, connecting through sight, sound, smell, and touch. In this sensory woodland walk you'll be focusing on each of your senses and what they are telling you. See them as antennae that collect information and help you build a three-dimensional picture of the environment. Take your time; allow yourself the opportunity to absorb every detail.

Once you've decided on a location for your ramble, make sure you are wearing the right clothes and footwear. The weather may be dry, but be aware that you may stumble on some mossy, muddy patches as you walk, so wear sensible shoes that support your ankles. Also, the weather in autumn can be unpredictable, so it's always useful to keep a waterproof with you, even if you don't need it when you first venture out.

Before you set off, check your route online or with a map, so you know where you are heading.

STEP 1 *As you walk, introduce each of your senses gradually,* by identifying things that you can see, hear, smell, and touch. For example, first you might notice the color palette—the rich array of hues and how the sun dances lightly on the fallen leaves.

STEP 2 *Take a moment to formulate a sentence that describes what you see,* so you might say: "A blanket of russet and gold surrounds me." Be sure to focus on this image, so you can store it as a memory in your mind's eye.

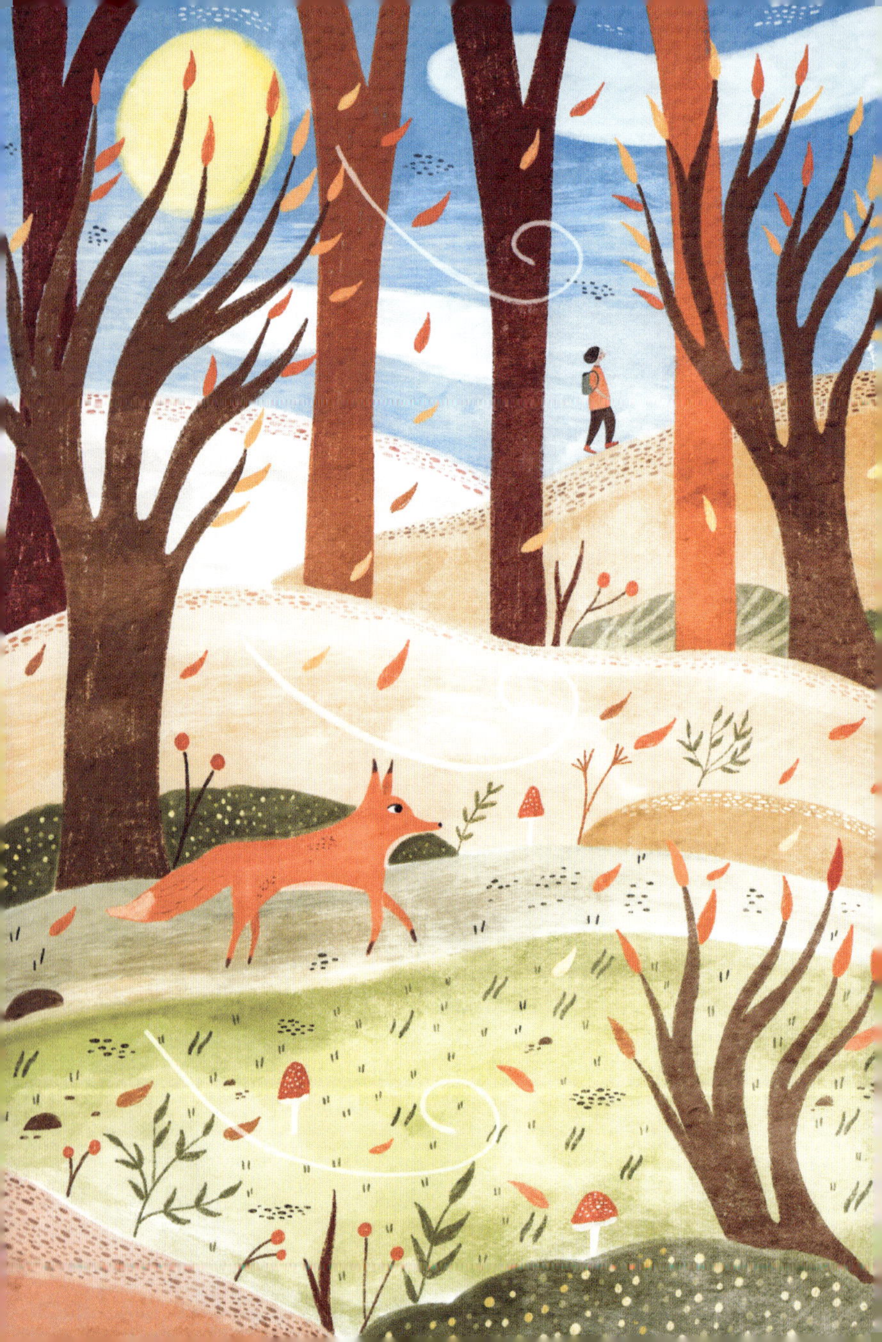

STEP 3 *Continue on your path and notice what you can hear*—perhaps the rustling of small animals in the undergrowth, a flutter of bird's wings, or the crackle and crunch of leaves underfoot. Highlight your favorite sound and describe it in your mind.

STEP 4 *Think about what you can smell*; for example, you might notice the earthy mustiness of fungi growing among the tree trunks, or the tinge of rain in the air. Again, isolate one thing that stands out, and come up with a description that captures the aroma.

STEP 5 *Consider what you feel as you meander in the woods*. You might notice that it is colder beneath the trees, or perhaps you feel a tingle of moisture on your face. Again, reflect on this, and the feeling that stands out the most, and sum it up in a few words. Take your time with each of these steps and really focus on each sensation and what it is that you like about it.

STEP 6 *Continue strolling through the woods,* engaging all of your senses at the same time. Notice how this brings the scenery to life in new ways.

WALK 4

Contrasting Amble

While some walkers prefer to explore new locations and change things up, there's something to be said for wandering down well-worn, familiar paths. The route may be recognizable, but that doesn't mean it can't surprise you.

Our surroundings change from day to day, and while it might not be as evident, over time and given the seasonal transitions, you'll begin to notice the impact of the elements and how regular routes are enhanced. If you look through fresh eyes, you'll appreciate the woods that you know well and be enchanted by the way they evolve through the year.

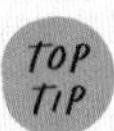

RECORD YOUR MEMORIES

Organize your thoughts, pictures, and reflections in a woodland journal. You can also include quotes, snippets of poems, sketches, and anything else that helps you bring each season to life. If you walk as a family, your children might enjoy getting involved and helping you create a book that charts the seasonal changes in their favorite woods. Encourage them to stretch their imagination and get creative with each entry.

SEASONAL SNAPSHOT

Each transitional shift brings its own magic. You may have your favorites, but this could change as you move through the year. The key is to have a pictorial record of your woodland walks, so that you can reflect upon them at the end of the year and recognize the beauty of each season.

Use a phone or other camera to record the same woodland walk in a series of snapshots, which you will then replicate at different times during the year. The ultimate goal is to collect a selection of shots of the same spots in spring, summer, autumn, and winter, so you can see each season's influence clearly.

STEP 1 *To begin, identify your markers,* the points along the route where you want to take your pictures. These have to be identical for each woodland walk and taken from the same perspective. For example, you might pick an ancient oak, and if you take the picture looking up into the boughs of the tree, then you would need to take it from that viewpoint each time. Make sure your markers are things that remain whatever time of year it is.

STEP 2 *When you have finished,* save the photographs either on your phone or computer; alternatively, you may want to print them off and keep them in a journal.

STEP 3 *At the end of the year,* reflect upon your artistic endeavors. Which photographs appeal and why? What is it about the season that strikes a chord with you? Have your opinions changed? For example, you might not be a fan of the colder, harsher conditions of winter, but on reflection you can see the starkly beautiful effect it has on the landscape.

WALK 5

Soothe with Shinrin-yoku

Originating in Japan in the early 1980s, the practice of forest bathing, also known as Shinrin-yoku, was first introduced by the government as part of a national health program to alleviate depression, lower stress levels, and improve concentration and creativity. It is about being mindfully aware as you stand or walk in nature, with the intention of breathing in the tranquility of the landscape.

Today it is a wellness staple, and a popular way to boost the mood. Based on the Shinto principle that nature is sacred and good for body, mind, and soul, forest bathing schools and guided walks are available throughout the world. Wherever there's a patch of woodland, there's the potential to luxuriate in the joy of flora and fauna, using mindful techniques.

FOREST BATHING WALK

Forest bathing is about taking in every aspect of your surroundings, being present in the moment, and breathing in the beauty. It's important to take the time to reflect on your journey, to process everything you see and feel, and let the entire experience envelop you in calmness.

STEP 1 *Before you enter the woodland area, take a moment to still your heart and mind.* Take a long, deep breath in, drawing it through the soles of your feet, up along your legs, and into your torso. Feel the breath settle in the center of your chest and hold it there for a count of four.

STEP 2 *Exhale, and let the breath filter out slowly between your lips.* As you do this, focus on your feet and how they anchor you to the ground. Feel that connection and know that you are supported by the earth as you walk.

STEP 3 *Begin to take a steady stroll through the woods.* Adopt a slow, gradual pace, and concentrate on the feel of the land and navigating the path.

STEP 4 *Each time you inhale, imagine you are drawing in the stillness of this place,* pulling it deep into your heart where it permeates you with peace. Allow the stillness to sit there for a moment. Don't be in a rush to exhale. Enjoy these long, slow breaths and know that every time you take one, you are being infused with the power of nature.

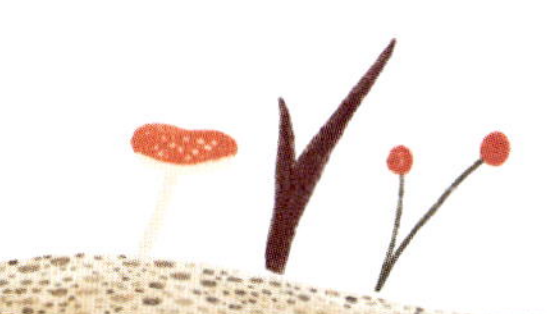

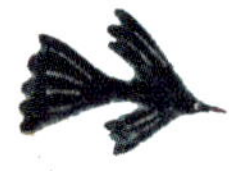

STEP 5 *As you release the breath,* imagine the forest drawing closer until it feels as if the leafy shrubs and towering trees have cocooned you in a cloak ofvegetation. Feel the damp air cling to your skin and know that it is simply the forest holding you in a welcoming and soothing embrace.

STEP 6 *Engage each of your senses as you walk.* Look at the colors and textures around you and don't be afraid to reach out: to feel the bark of the tree, to hold a leaf between your fingers and smell its sharp freshness. Take in every aspect of your environment.

STEP 7 *Pause when something captures your attention and lean into it.* Draw in the beauty and let the magic of this space lift your spirits. Say either out loud or in your head: "I am a part of nature and nature is a part of me."

STEP 8 *Enjoy the rest of the walk in this way,* and take note of your thoughts and feelings when you have finished your ramble.

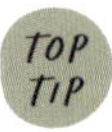

MAKE THE MOST OF YOUR EXPERIENCE

To make the most of a forest bathing walk, take a blanket with you and find somewhere to sit and really soak up the stillness. This could be at the base of a tree, on a tree stump, or in a patch of grass. If you're sitting on the ground, place both hands on either side, palms facing downward. Let your palms connect with the woodland floor. Don't be afraid to get soil between your fingers and really feel the earth on your skin. Close your eyes for a few seconds and focus on your breathing. Let the sounds and smells of nature fill you up. Then, when you're ready, take a moment to stretch and shake your limbs out after this brief sojourn and continue on your way.

WALK 6

Ignite Your Creative Spark

Studies show that taking a walk increases your creativity by up to sixty percent. It's thought that fresh air and natural light provide the optimum conditions for your brain to thrive. Combine this with the solitude and space that a stroll through the woods offers and you may find that the forest backdrop provides just the right balance of space and feel-good vibes to ignite that creative spark!

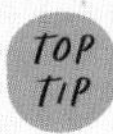

GROW YOUR OWN

Truly connect with the fertile and creative energy of the environment by doing some planting. Look around you at the plants and shrubs and how they create the beautiful setting that you are enjoying. Tap into this energy by planting up a pot with your choice of flower or herb, such as sweet-scented lavender. Add the right amount of potting compost to the pot, then use your hands to create a space for the fledgling plant. Gently secure the plant in place, using your fingertips to pat down the compost. As you do this, recognize that you are tapping into the creative force of nature that you have seen firsthand on your walk. Water well and place in a sunny location, ensuring the plant is somewhere easy for you to see. Watch and enjoy the plant's progress as it grows and flourishes.

AN ARTY AMBLE

Make the most of a woodland ramble by using the time to think creatively. Reduce your stress and disconnect from technology. It's time to go back to basics. Return to your childhood and give your brain time to breathe. In doing so, you'll allow your imagination to take over. You will need a notebook or journal, a pen, and a flask or bottle of water as you may be out for some time.

STEP 1 *Slow and steady is the key.* Creativity cannot be forced, but it can be directed and given the space to flourish. This walk is about providing that space and letting nature inspire you, so set a pace but take your time. Get into a rhythm, which can actually help your creative flow, and let the sounds of nature envelop you.

STEP 2 *Let your attention go where it needs to be.* For example, if the flutter of feathers against leaves makes you look up, follow the sound. If a fallen tree looks almost human in shape, spend some time taking it in, running your hand over the bark and observing it from all angles. Let your imagination take over and make narrative connections.

STEP 3 *Pause and reflect.* Creativity needs a starting point, something to trigger its flow, so it's important to allow those thoughts to surface. Take regular breaks along the path for pondering. Get out your notebook or journal and put pen to paper. Even if you feel your mind is blank, your latent creativity might surprise you with a doodle or a rhyme.

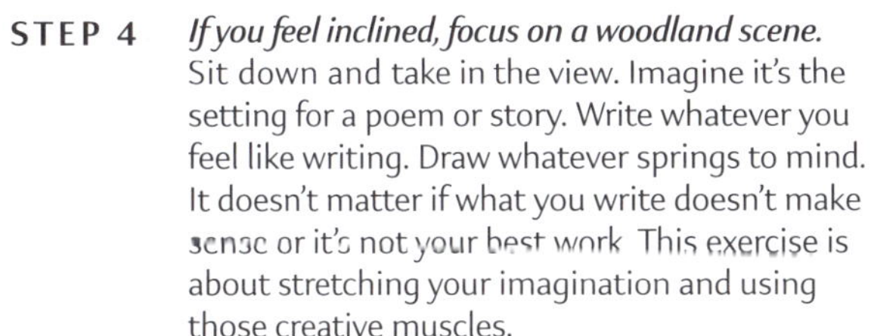

STEP 4 *If you feel inclined, focus on a woodland scene.* Sit down and take in the view. Imagine it's the setting for a poem or story. Write whatever you feel like writing. Draw whatever springs to mind. It doesn't matter if what you write doesn't make sense or it's not your best work. This exercise is about stretching your imagination and using those creative muscles.

STEP 5 *Rejoin the path* and redouble your creative efforts by taking your lead from Mother Nature. Consider how the woods have evolved over time, how the path you walk winds in different directions, and how the shrubs and trees have always taken hold and shaped the landscape.

STEP 6 *After your walk,* take a moment to reflect upon the experience and look at your creative output. Even if you have struggled to produce anything on paper, you might find that your head is full of ideas and your mind is open and ready for action.

WALK 7

Go on Safari

A woodland safari is an exciting experience and something you can do easily on your regular walks. You will need appropriate clothing, a pair of binoculars, a notepad to record any special sightings, and some refreshments. The woods are rich with diversity, from plants and trees to an array of mammals, insects, and birds, so you're bound to find something that piques your interest!

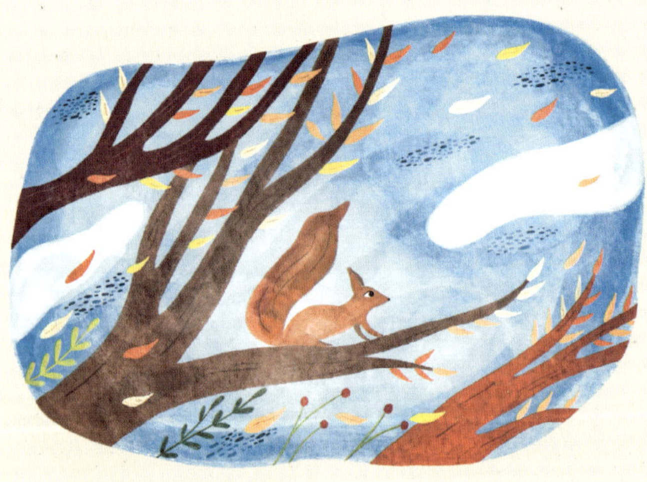

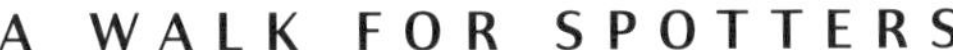

A WALK FOR SPOTTERS

You'll need a keen eye and lots of patience for this type of walk. The key is to stay present, in the moment, and pay attention. Here are some tips to help you get the most out of your day.

- You'll be spotting as you stroll, so engage all your senses and take your time.
- Have a location in mind roughly halfway through the walk where you can sit in the undergrowth and observe your surroundings for a short while. If you do this, you're likely to see more creatures going about their daily business.
- Look from all angles. Don't stick to what is directly ahead of you: look down at your feet and you might notice animal tracks; look up in the air and you will see birds in flight.
- Study the trees. There's a lot of activity in a single tree, from insects and birds that live in the trunk or perch on the branches, to creatures like squirrels who hop and jump around the leafy canopy.
- Look beneath stones and dead wood. Don't ignore fallen pieces of wood, tree stumps, or rocks; be curious and take a look underneath, and you will discover an entire ecosystem. Always return things to their original state, as you don't want to disturb any wildlife that you find.

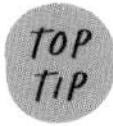

FAMILY FUN

A safari walk is a great activity for younger members of the family, so get them on board. Make a day of it and take a picnic with you. Have fun and see who can find the largest range of insects, birds, mammals, and so on.

WALK 8

Wander Through the Wildflowers

A wide range of wildflowers can be found in woodlands around the world. Wildflower diversity peaks and dips, depending on the type of bloom, climate, and location. Shade-tolerant plants like delicate bluebells do well in dense, leafy areas, but other, rarer species may struggle. Even so, there is much to discover on a woodland walk, if you're prepared to look beneath the surface.

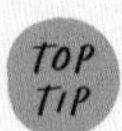

THE WISDOM OF FLOWERS

Keep a journal of your woodland walk and use it to record the different flowers and herbs you find. When you get home, spend some time learning about your discoveries. There are so many herbs and blooms around the world that you'll find a wealth of interesting facts, some based on superstition and others on a flower's traditional uses, be those medicinal or practical. Reading more about the botanical features of different blooms will help you to recognize and appreciate their presence the next time you go on a woodland ramble.

WILDFLOWER WALK

Your observations skills will be put to the test on this kind of walk. You need to pay attention and actively seek out herbs and flowers hidden in the undergrowth. It helps if you have an identification app on your phone or a guidebook to help you pinpoint which type of bloom it is. A little background research on the season and location is also helpful; consider the time of year and which species are likely to be in flower.

- A wildflower walk can help you connect with the landscape at a deeper level. Like any mindful activity, you'll need to engage your senses, paying attention to what you see and smell.
- Enjoy the walk as you would usually, but stay present by focusing on the smaller details: the plants and leaves at your feet, the clumps hidden behind tree stumps, and the climbers that trail around tree trunks or along the forest floor.
- Follow your nose and let the sweet herbal aromas lead you to your destination. Once you've discovered what you think is a flower or herb, it's time to identify it!

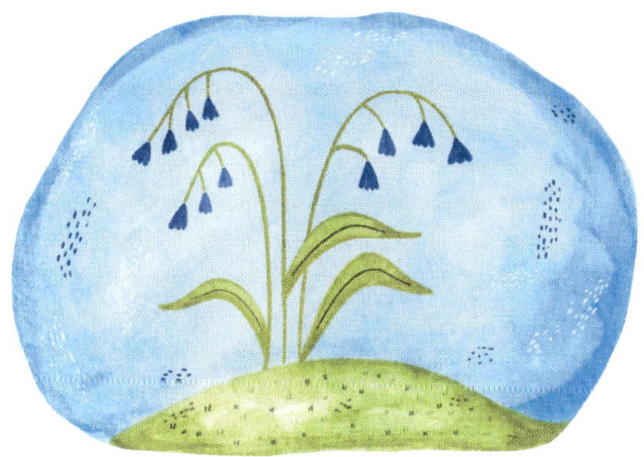

WILDFLOWER CHECKLIST

This quick guide outlines what you need to look for when identifying blooms.

- Start from the base of the stem and work your way up. Look at the stem: is it one solid stalk, or are there many? Do the shoots spread across the floor or stand erect? Is the stem tall or small and stocky?
- Check out the size and shape of the leaves. Are they large or small? Broad or narrow? Do they fan out or are they pointed? Also consider the texture: are they smooth or hairy? Do they feel waxy to the touch or have a rich sheen? What about the color?
- Look at the flower heads. How big are they? Wildflowers tend to be smaller and often grow in abundance. What kind of shape are the flowers? Do they look like a daisy or are they more bell-shaped? How many petals and sepals do the flowers have?
- Consider the color of the flowers. Wildflowers come in a variety of hues, and some even have patterns.
- Finally, engage your sense of smell. Do the flowers have a scent, and if so, what does it remind you of?

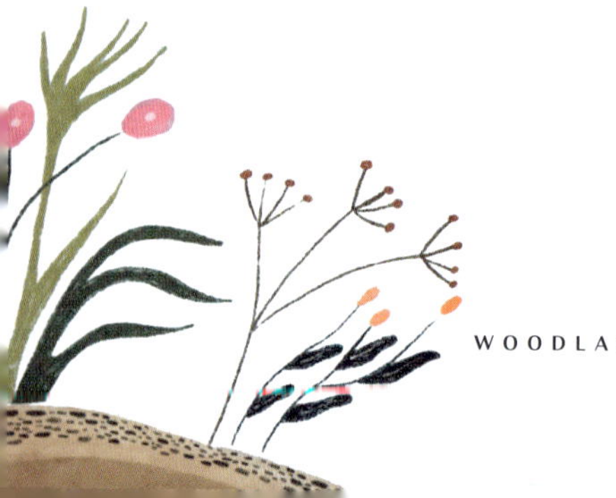

WALK 9

Lose Yourself in the Magic

In folklore people would go to the woods for spiritual sustenance and to perform rituals to help them harness natural power. There are many traditions throughout mythology, which are rooted in forest lore. Norse mythology describes how the god Odin spent nine days and nights hanging from Yggdrasil—a giant ash tree. The sap from the branches sustained him as he searched for sacred knowledge. The Sun Dance of the Indigenous Americans of the Great Plains features a pole from a cottonwood tree, symbolizing the connection to the Great Spirit. The Celts created their own rituals, tying rags to low-hanging tree branches as a way of petitioning the gods. You may not follow the old ways, but there is still much here to help you feel inspired and reconnect with nature.

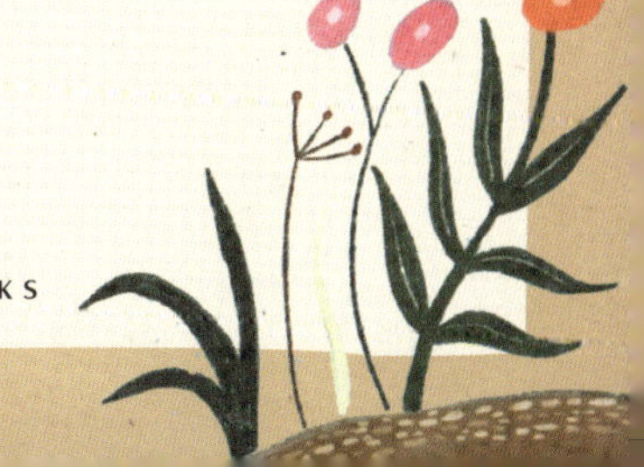

RITUAL RAMBLE

Adopt a magical approach to your next woodland ramble, and use the time to reflect upon your hopes and dreams, by adapting a Celtic custom and making it your own. Take a small piece of ribbon with you in whatever color you like. If you want to write something down, take a pen and some paper too.

STEP 1 *Find a place you know well,* so choose a walk you have done before and that you enjoy. You might already have a favorite spot along your route, but if not, simply enjoy wandering the path until you come to a space that feels special to you.

STEP 2 *Sit or stand in this space and take in its beauty.* Breathe deeply and feel infused by the energy of the woods. Think about your hopes and dreams for the future and what would make you happy, and let those thoughts play out in your head. Let your imagination take over and daydream a little.

STEP 3 *Find a low-hanging branch in the vicinity* and tie the ribbon to one of its twigs. You don't need a lot of ribbon for this. The idea is that the ribbon anchors you to nature and connects you with the creative power of the Earth. Alternatively, if you prefer, you can write a wish on a small piece of paper, then fold it up tightly and, using your hands, bury it as deep as you can in the soil.

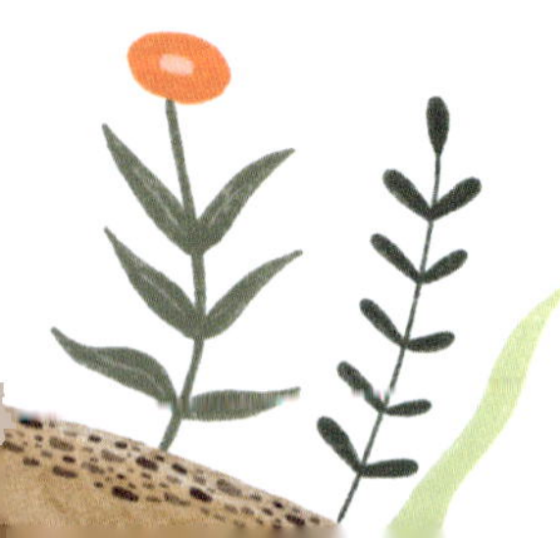

STEP 4 *Sit for a minute with those hopes and dreams.* Imagine how you'll feel when they come true and enjoy reveling in those positive emotions. Let the fertile spirit of the woods excite you about the future. After all, you are a part of nature and have the same creative ability at your fingertips, which means you have the power to manifest positive change! When you are ready, leave the space and continue on your path. Be sure to breathe, relax, and enjoy the rest of your walk.

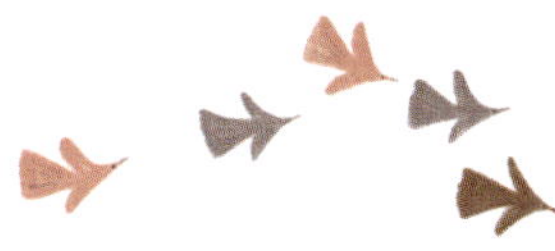

TRY THIS

A NATURAL KEEPSAKE

To reinforce your connection with the woodland, and cement your ritual, you might want to take a memento with you. Choose something small and easy to carry, something that won't be missed and will not cause any harm to the environment, such as a stone, feather, leaf, or acorn. Keep the memento in your hands or pocket as you finish your stroll, and then store it somewhere safe at home, so you can be reminded of the ritual walk and what it means to you.

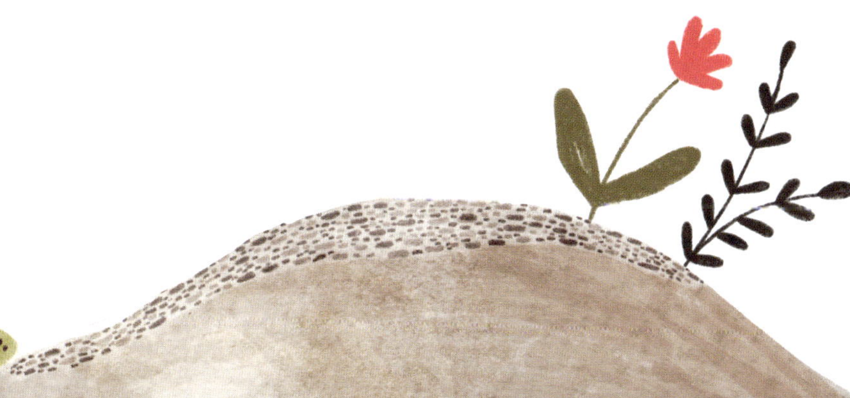

WALK 10

Wander and Ponder

A brisk woodland walk during the chillier months is good for your health! Not only does the cold air slow down the growth of bacteria, it is also a great way to boost the immune system. Exposure to colder temperatures increases the number of white blood cells that fight infection.

Combine this with the mental benefits of fresh air, a stirringly beautiful backdrop sprinkled with frost and ice, and the opportunity to observe wildlife clearly, thanks to bare branches and tracks in the snow, and there's no excuse not to don your winter woollies and get outside!

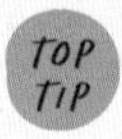

FEEL YOUR WAY

Engage your sense of touch. It may be cold outside, but make the most of the refreshing energy that a drop in temperature brings. Bend down and touch the earth, feel the icy frost on your fingertips, and how it makes the ground smooth. Let your hand glide across the trunk of your favorite tree. How does it feel? It will be a different experience from earlier in the year, when the bark was warmed by the sun. Feel the earth beneath your boots as you walk. Let your weight fall into your heels and toes, so your steps are springy and supercharged with energy.

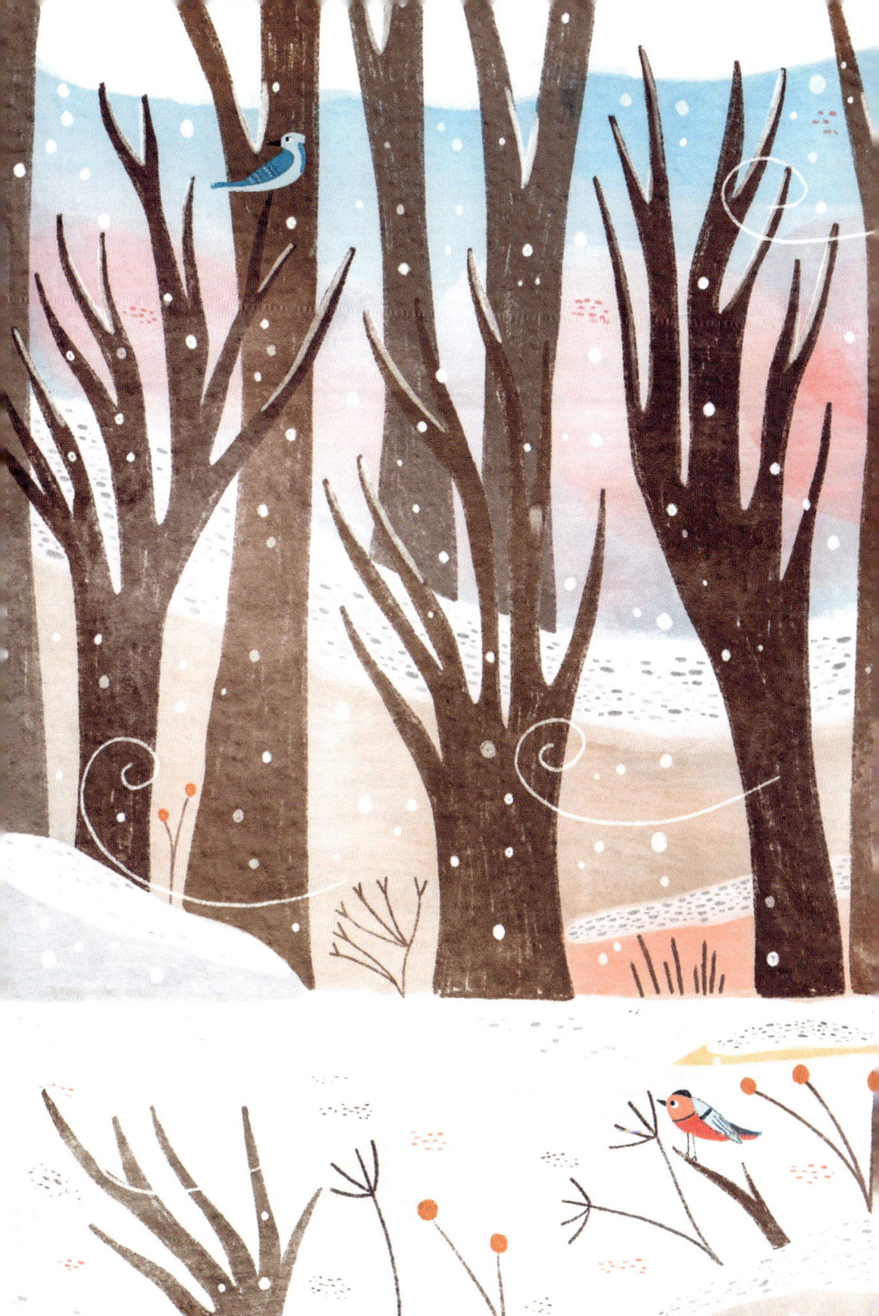

A "GO WITHIN" WALK

During the colder months, the woods become a winter wonderland, a glistening vision punctuated by the bareness of the trees. The landscape may feel empty in places, but there is much joy to be had in a winter stroll, especially if you use the time to engage, reflect, and recharge.

Before you begin, wrap up in plenty of layers, including waterproofs, and ensure you have the right shoes or boots to cope with slippery, cold surfaces underfoot. You're going to be walking at a brisk pace to keep warm, so you need to be sure-footed!

STEP 1 *Choose a path that you have walked before*, so you are accustomed to your surroundings and the route. Let the rhythm of your stride and your confident gait push you onward. Let this focus your mind as you stroll.

STEP 2 *Listen to the sound of your feet* crunching along the path and observe the changes underfoot too, such as the tiny markings left by the birds and any other animal tracks that catch your eye. Feel the crisp chill of the air against your cheeks. Let the cold enliven your senses.

STEP 3 *Take short, sharp, deep breaths* in time with your footfall. Feel the cold air inflate your lungs and clear your head, providing the focus and clarity you need to go within.

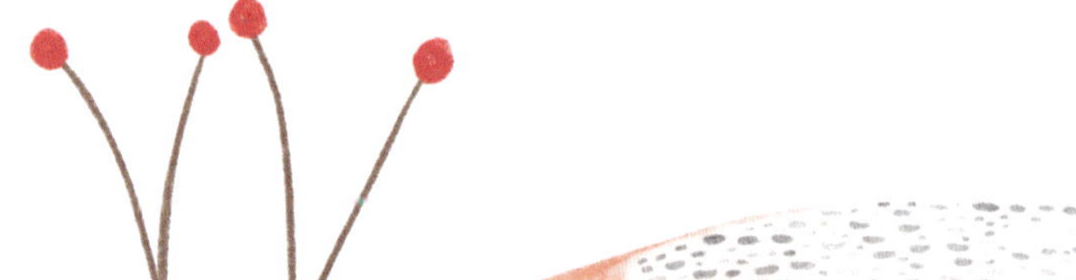

STEP4 *Think back through the events of the year* as you walk. Consider each challenge, each triumph, each achievement, however big or small, and recognize their worth. Know that you have done your best, and acknowledge this with every step.

STEP 5 *Enjoy the pace of the walk* and notice the stark, brittle surroundings. Appreciate the way the trees look familiar but different and how they have adapted in order to survive and thrive. Know that as you walk into the winter months, you too will adapt and go with the flow. You will appreciate the benefits of the season.

STEP 6 *Feel a sense of accomplishment* as you get closer to your destination.

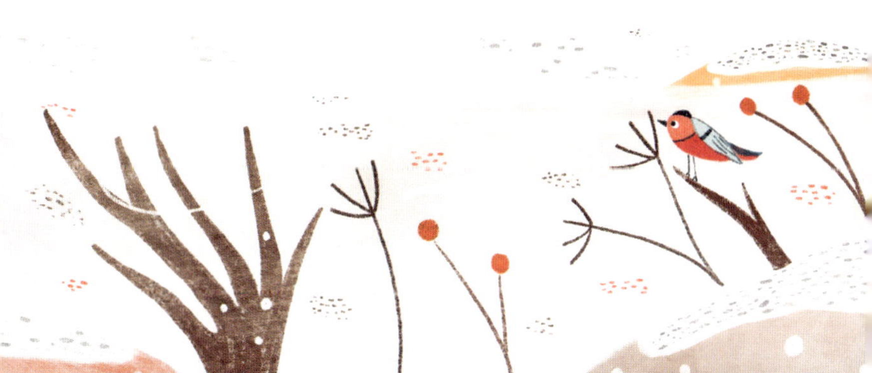

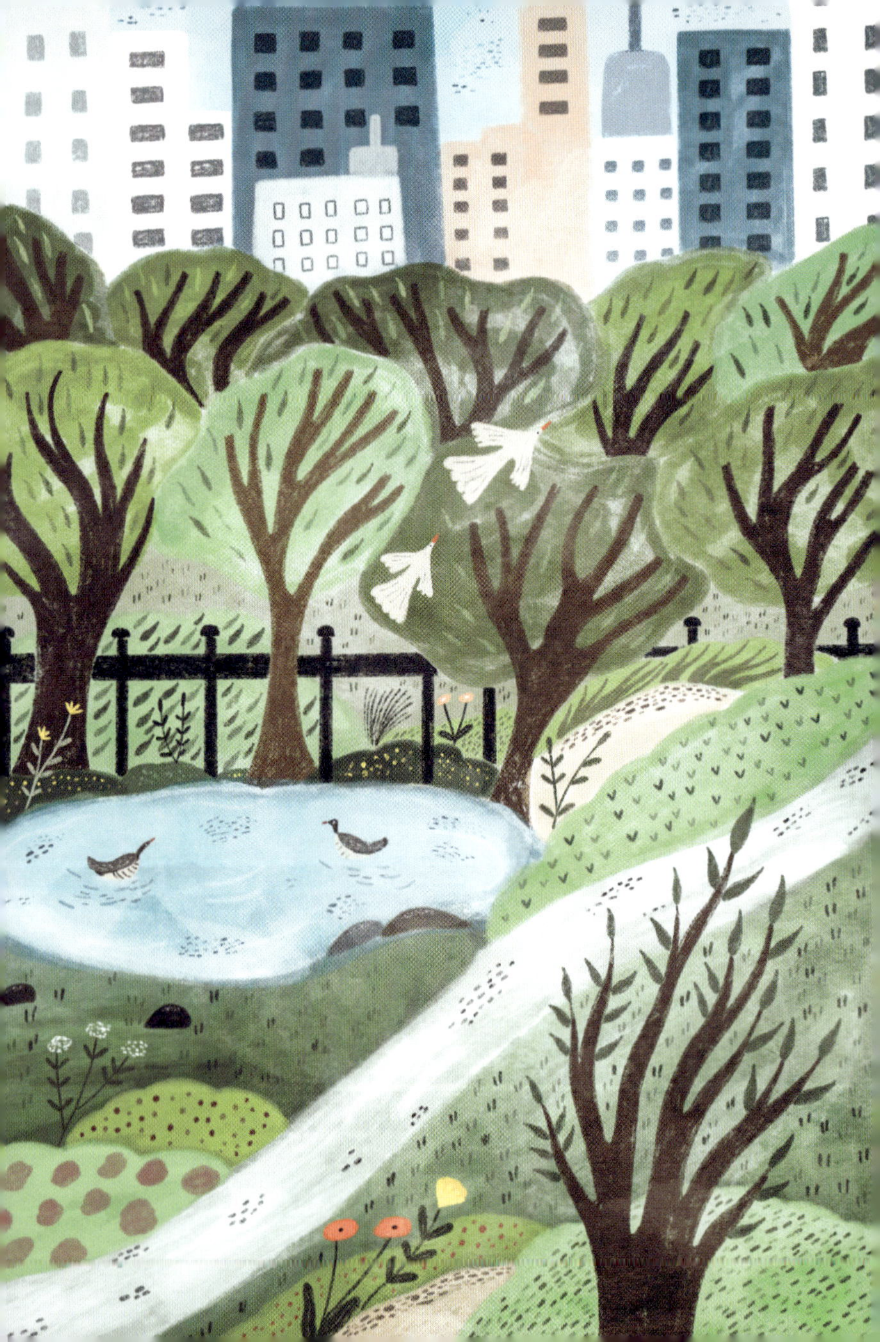

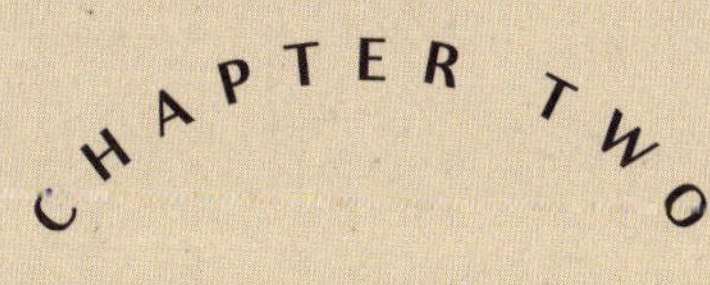

Urban Walks

Cityscapes have much to offer, especially for those who seek stimulation. You may be walking solo, but you're not actually on your own—you are part of a community. And if you really want to get to know a place, then the only way to do this is on foot.

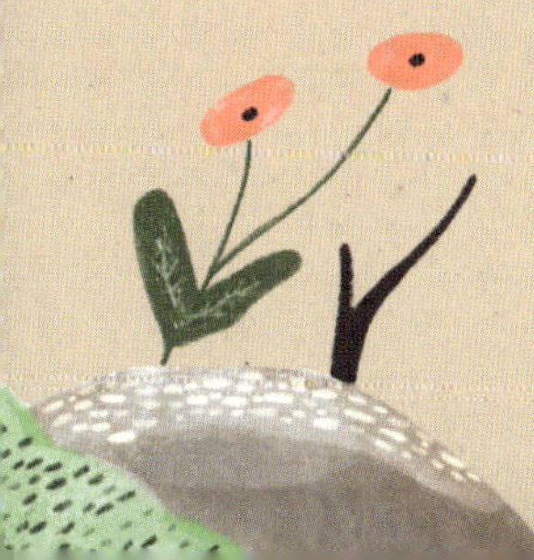

WALK 11

Conquer the Urban Maze

Serendipity plays a role in urban walking. There's the opportunity to learn and discover, to let intuition take the lead and seize the moment by taking a new turn, which might reveal something that you never knew existed. Even dead-ends have their beauty, giving the urban landscape the mystery of a concrete maze. Every avenue directs you to your destination and a new adventure. You're also less likely to get lost in a city as there are always landmarks and people on hand to help. This alone makes detours and flights of fancy possible.

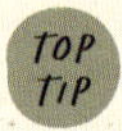

SHARE THE EXPERIENCE

If you enjoy your solo adventure, why not take a friend next time? Another person will have a different perspective and will notice things that you miss, so their input can enrich the experience. Exploring something together is a lot of fun; it gives you time to truly connect with your companion and learn something new about them.

URBAN RAMBLING

Get to know your city with an off-the-cuff ramble that takes you out of your comfort zone and into pastures new! Revel and reflect in the beauty of your city, by setting yourself a walking challenge that will broaden your horizons.

Take a bus or the subway to the outskirts of the city, to somewhere you don't know, then work your way back to the center. All you need is a sense of adventure, comfy walking shoes, and plenty of time. This is not something you can do in a limited time period; this is about moving freely in your space and going with the flow of urban life.

- It helps if you have a rough idea of the direction you'll be traveling, but there's no need to plan your excursion to the letter. This is about having an adventure and seeking out paths that you wouldn't usually follow.
- Remember that you can follow signs and use a map or navigation tool on your phone if you feel the need, or simply go with the flow, letting your intuition and word of mouth lead you onwards.
- Have fun exploring. If you see something you like, stop and take a closer look. If you're drawn down a road that isn't taking you to your final destination, don't worry. You're allowed to go off the beaten track and satisfy your curiosity, so check out that local park or city garden if it piques your interest.
- Engage your senses as you walk. Think about what you can see, hear, smell, and feel.
- Give yourself plenty of time for this, so you can relax and have a real adventure. By doing so, you'll discover that the place you thought you knew has so much more to offer.

WALK 12

Pound the Pavements

You might think city streets offer little to excite the mind. The sidewalk, whether uniform or uneven, is just a concrete walkway and a means of getting from A to B. However, even if the landscape is bland, the connection you form with the path that you walk can make a huge difference to how you feel. By shifting your perspective, you can bring the experience of walking the same route to life in new and engaging ways.

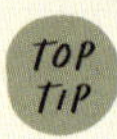

CREATE YOUR OWN SOUNDTRACK

Combine the rhythm of your feet with some powerful affirmations to make the most of your walk. For example, if you'd like to feel energized, you could create a positive statement that embodies this, such as: "I am brimming with energy," or "I am energized." Then repeat this phrase in your head as you walk, timing it to fit in with each beat. If you prefer, you could simply focus on the word "energy" and what this means. Imagine being infused with energy as you walk, and increase the power of your steps and rhythm to promote this further. Remember, you are creating the soundtrack to your walk, so you can incorporate any movement or sound you like to enhance this.

FOOT-DRUMMING WALK

Combine the senses of hearing and feeling with your body's natural rhythm to develop your own urban-based symphony as you walk. It might sound complicated, but all it takes is a little awareness of the impact that you make as you connect with your environment and the imprint you leave.

STEP 1 *Begin your walk as you would normally, but focus on the lower half of your body* and the gentle rhythm that you make as you take each step.

STEP 2 *Bring your attention to the sole of each foot*, and how it feels when you connect with the sidewalk beneath you, starting with your heel and rolling toward your toe.

STEP 3 *Notice the sound that your feet make* as they hit the sidewalk. Is it an obvious thwack, a light tap, or a deeper thrum? Does the sound change depending on the surface you are walking on?

STEP 4 *Begin to tap out a rhythm* by counting each step and feeling it resonate through your body. Experiment by changing the pace or putting more effort into your steps. Think of yourself as a musical artist composing your own theme tune as you walk.

STEP 5 *You may find that there are natural breaks*, times when you pause or the rhythm changes—this is all part of the symphony that you are creating.

STEP 6 *Enjoy the experience and have fun* switching things up by adding in more footsteps or even lengthening your stride. Know that even the dullest walk can provide an opportunity for you to be creative.

WALK 13

Switch It Up

Walking isn't just about countryside hikes or strolling by the sea. Every day provides the opportunity to get out and about into the fresh air and enjoy some exercise.

Studies show that a daily ten-minute walk lowers blood pressure and improves cholesterol levels, which in turn promotes heart health. It also contributes to the recommended 150 minutes of physical activity that every adult should aim to achieve each week, so, while a casual stroll to and from the store can become routine, it's still very much a game-changer when it comes to health and switching up the mindset.

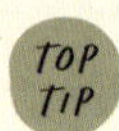

CHANGE YOUR ROUTINE

Walking at different times of the day changes your experience, so if you usually take a lunchtime saunter, mix things up and try the same route early in the morning; or, if you're a morning walker, go later in the day when there's more activity. You will notice new things, which will enhance your walk.

LOOK WITH FRESH EYES

When you only have time for a short walk you can't go far, but there's still plenty of potential for fun. Your usual patch may be well trodden and familiar, especially if it's a journey you do every day like a brisk commute to and from work, but that doesn't mean it can't be an engaging experience.

As you step out onto the street, imagine you're a tourist in your own world. This is the first time you have seen this vista, so everything is new to you. While this might take a leap of imagination, once you start looking at things through fresh eyes you will notice so much more, and this will enrich the experience. To help, follow these easy steps.

STEP 1 *Start with your breath.* Take a slow, deep breath in through your nose and then exhale gently through pursed lips. As you do this, notice what you can smell. You might pick up the scent of the trees and bushes that line the streets, or the aroma of freshly cut grass from lawns and roadsides. Have you noticed this before or is this something totally new?

STEP 2 *Focus on what you can see.* Try and pick out something that you haven't noticed before. For example, you may spot a cut-through that you've always missed, or a pretty shrub in bloom. Look for things that usually pass you by and make a mental note of them.

STEP 3 *Acknowledge the usual everyday sights that greet you,* but take your time and look at them from a different perspective, such as the slope of the street and how it curves into a beautiful arch, and how this might look from a distance; the way a tree by the intersection towers above you, providing shelter in all types of weather, its gnarled branches stretching in every direction like a spider's web. Look at things from alternative angles to gain a fuller picture. Enjoy picking out objects of interest and engaging with them in a new way.

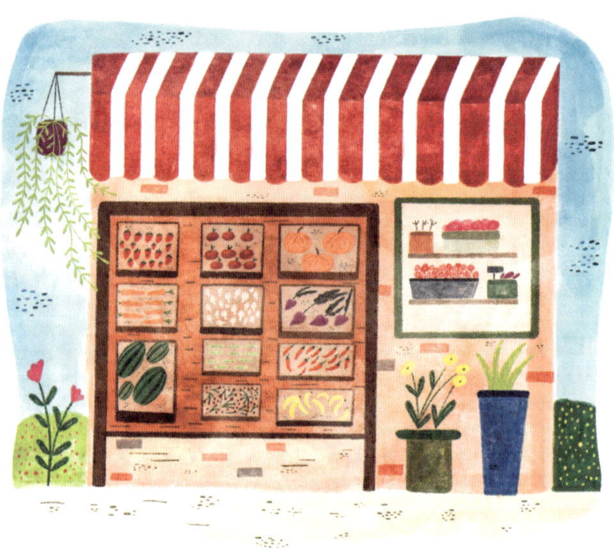

WALK 14

Wake Up with the City

There is nothing like an early morning urban stroll to cleanse body, mind, and soul. Watching the day unfold is a powerful experience. Those first stirrings, when movement is slow and slumbering, give you time to adjust to the world, to truly breathe in your surroundings and appreciate the clean slate of a new day.

Daylight emerges gradually; it doesn't charge ahead with bluster, bullying the nocturnal hours into submission. It glides with all the grace of a ballerina, gently taking center stage—a dawn stroll should be the same. Harness the stillness of this transitional time and let your body and mind acclimatize.

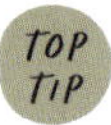

WRITE YOUR OWN STORY

Be your own narrator. To help you on your morning ambles, you might want to record a guided visualization that you can listen to as you walk. You could take inspiration from the heavens, or come up with your own adapted version. There are plenty of guided visualizations available online that you can use or tweak to suit your needs.

If you're feeling really creative, take your walk with the intention of creating a narrative to go with it, something that you can reflect upon and record later in the day. To help, make some notes, either in a notebook or on your phone, of things that you see and how they make you feel. You are the author of your own story and you know what inspires you, so focus on the things that lift your mood.

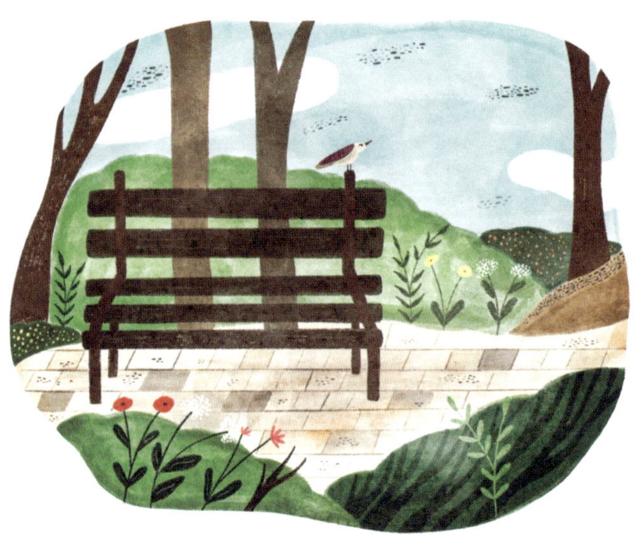

PICTURE THIS

A dawn walk in the city is calm and liberating. The energy is different, slow, steady, but also bristling with potential. This is the perfect time to contemplate, to mull over your aspirations and the passions that drive you onward. Take inspiration from your surroundings. Whether you're strolling along the empty streets, drifting past sleepy houses, or taking a meander through the park, embrace the tranquility and know that each new day provides the opportunity to try again, to create something new.

- Let your imagination flow. Allow daydreams to command your senses: there is no need to rush, you have all the time in the world at this moment. What do you most want from today? How would you like things to go? Let your emotions pick up speed, as the world begins to move around you.

- Hear the birds' morning song bright and cheerful in your ears as you stroll. See this song as a call to arms, nature's way of heralding a new beginning. See the concrete jungle slowly come to life, as streets are swept and cars begin their steady crawl forward, and know that it is time to go with the tide, to give your dreams wings and watch them take flight.

- Use this time to picture what you'd like to happen, today, tomorrow, and well into the future. Build those hopes in your mind and then see them emerge like a movie on a screen in your head that you can replay as you walk. Don't worry if other sights and sounds draw you away, as the joy of a morning stroll is in the lingering, the leisurely gait that allows you time to relax and visualize.

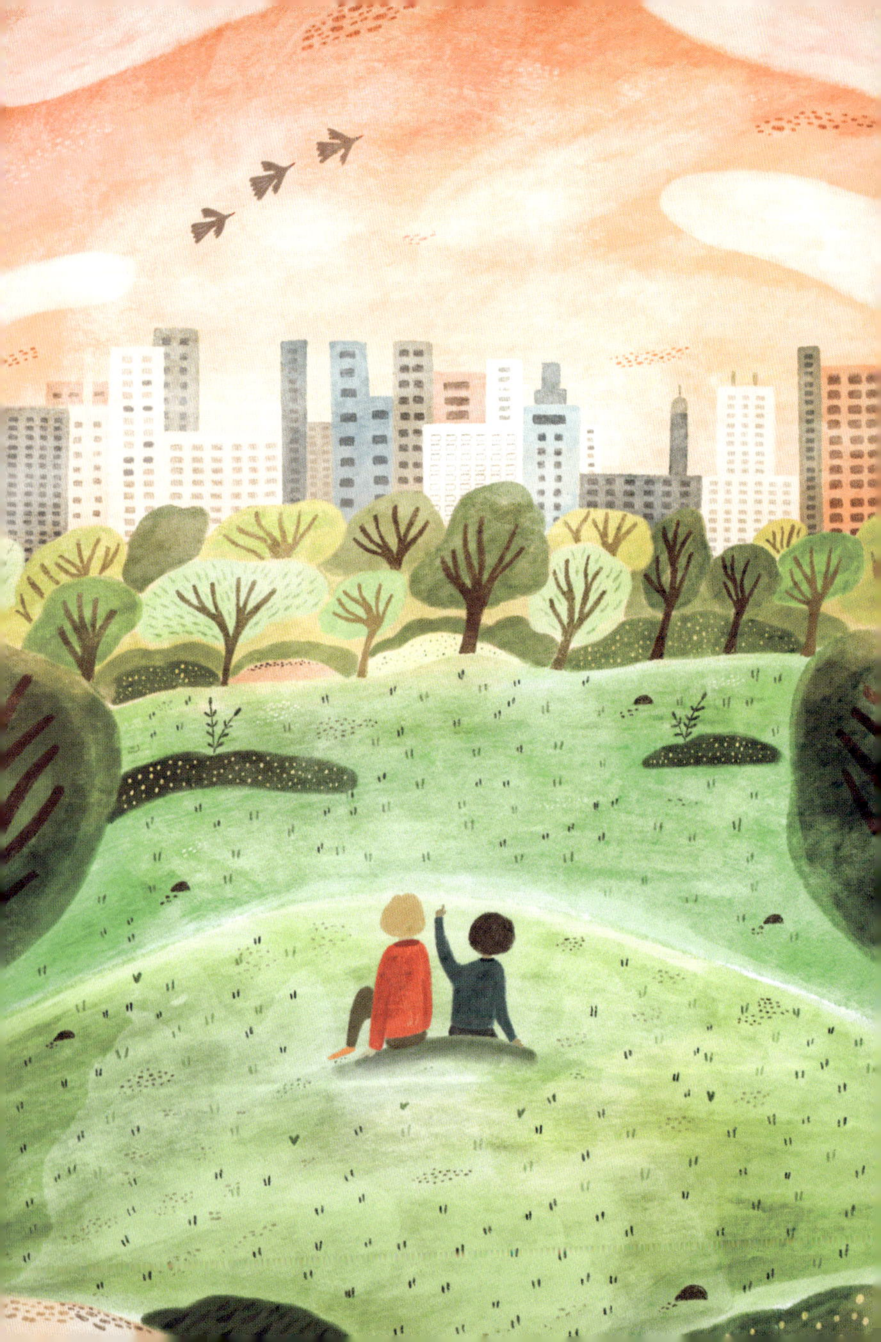

- Engage with your environment, and allow the slow awakening motivate you. Perhaps the slight circular swell on the surface of the pond as you walk by causes an internal ripple, an idea that comes from nowhere but begins to form a wave of excitement in your mind. Maybe the pigeons that peck hopefully beneath a park bench make you smile and remind you that there is no harm in trying, in asking for what you want and persevering with those dreams that you dismissed so quickly yesterday. After all, today is a new day and you are here, walking your walk, moving with the wheel of time and at the brink of your potential.

- You might want to pick up pace and be proactive in your thinking, seeking even more inspiration from the sights and sounds that greet you. Feel the sun's warmth on the top of your head and acknowledge that it too has turned up its shine in readiness for the unfolding day. Maybe it's a cold winter's morning and all you feel is the bitter chill of the wind whipping at your cheeks. Even so, there is still a message here, a sign of encouragement in the way the wind bites at your heels, pushing you onward. The fresh air fills your lungs with sustenance, powering those passions that are now overflowing and making every part of your body tingle with anticipation.

- The experience of a morning stroll will differ greatly depending on the season, but the theme is always the same. It is a fresh start, a new adventure, and you have taken the first step along the path. Keep going, keep moving, however slowly. Enjoy the stillness, the pause, and then the shift into activity as the morning unfurls like a beautiful flower.

WALK 15

Revel in Nature

The city is alive and thriving with nature, from roadside verges littered with wildflowers to abundant hedgerows fizzing with activity. Flowers peek from walled gardens and sidewalk strips house pretty displays that add a splash of brightness to the vista. Green space comes in many shapes and forms, with city parks and municipal gardens taking center stage for those who want to go off the beaten track, or need their nature fix. These mainstays wait patiently for us to discover their beauty. Whether recent additions or a hundred-year sentinels, these community hubs are perfect for those seeking the solace of flora and fauna in the midst of a busy schedule.

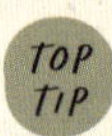

FAST-FORWARD

If you're pushed for time, you can still enjoy the benefits of a brisk walk. Regard this as a challenge to see and experience as much nature as you can, while walking at speed. Imagine the landscape wrapping around you as you step out. See it cloaking you in color and energy, then visualize it trailing behind you, as you walk.

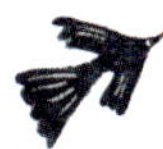

CAMERA ROLL WALK

City walks are often something you squeeze into your schedule, but that doesn't mean you can't reap the same benefits. Make the most of the time you have in the middle of a busy day by taking a short nature walk in your city park or gardens. Open your heart and mind and observe your surroundings from every angle to gain a fresh perspective and uncover hidden gems within your reach.

STEP 1 *Before you begin, set an intention with a positive affirmation* such as, "I am open and ready to connect with nature and absorb all the benefits of this green space."

STEP 2 *Gaze with purpose as you walk along, actively seeking things of beauty*. Imagine you're recording everything and your eyes are a camera, and take it all in. Notice the colors, the shapes, and the textures. For example, you might not usually pay much attention to the grass at your feet, but today make it the star of the show. Notice the bright green glimmer of each blade, the length of it, and the way the hues vary depending on the sunlight. You might spot a tiny beetle making its way through the undergrowth, or a beautiful butterfly sunning itself on a patch of grass.

STEP 3 *Be sure to look up too.* Instead of focusing solely on what is at eye level, cast your net wider. Gaze upward to the sky and look at the clouds and the shapes they make. Notice how fast they seem to be moving.

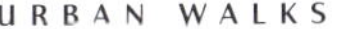

Look at the canopy of trees and take in the pattern of the branches. Notice the way they move in the breeze and the creatures that inhabit this space. Pick out the birds and watch them in flight.

STEP 4 *Engage your other senses to help you spot wildlife along the way.* For example, you might hear a snippet of birdsong, which would normally stay on the periphery of your mind. Today make this your focus and follow the sound. See where it leads and if you can spot the feathery performer.

STEP 5 *Stand for a moment and observe the view from every angle.* Spin around slowly to take it all in. Imagine you're filming this circular shot and commit as much detail as you can to memory, so you can call on it anytime you feel stressed. Breathe deeply and absorb the energy of this space. Let your body and mind recharge as you walk.

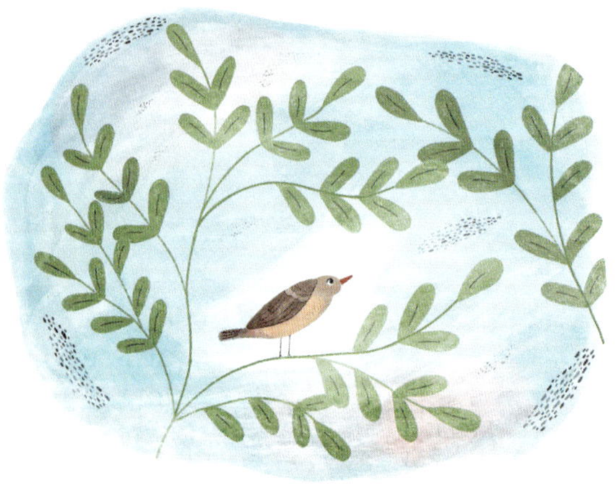

WALK 16

Give Your Brain a Workout

Studies show that walking at regular intervals throughout the week can boost cognitive function and enhance memory. Brisk exercise, which also stimulates problem-solving skills, promotes blood flow to the brain, which encourages the growth of cells in the hippocampus, the region responsible for memory and learning. In other words, a ten-minute stroll through the city can kick-start your gray matter, so you're firing on all cylinders for the rest of the day!

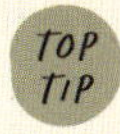

MAPPING YOUR MEMORIES

Instead of creating a memory walk by placing items or numbers from a list at different locations, why not try actual memories that bring you joy. For example, favorite moments from childhood, or special events and occasions that always make you smile. You can use people too. If there's someone who always lifts your spirits, bring their face to mind and position them at a key location on your walk, so you always think of them, or bring that specific memory to mind when you reach the same point on your route.

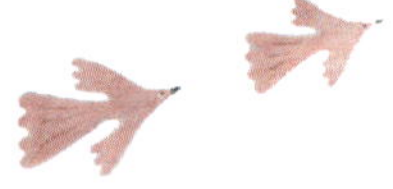

A MEMORY WALK

To further enhance the brain-boosting capabilities of an urban stroll, try this simple exercise, which stretches the imagination and helps to exercise your memory-building skills. The cityscape is the ideal backdrop for this, as you will find it easy to pick out the key focal points that form the basis of this technique.

It's a good idea to have a specific walk in mind for this that you do often—for example, your daily commute to and from the office might take you on a well-trodden path that you instinctively know, making it the ideal choice to engage your brain. You will need a list of items that you would like to recall in order, such as a series of digits that make up a telephone number or a shopping list.

STEP 1 *Begin your walk as you would normally,* making sure that you are relaxed by breathing properly. Focus on what you can see, feel, hear, and smell. Instead of letting thoughts come and go in your mind, concentrate on the list that you need to remember.

STEP 2 *As you walk, take note of your surroundings* and pick out key landmarks that catch your eye. For example, as you begin, you might walk past a canal that leads into the city and see a colorful barge that is there every day; this might be your first landmark. As you progress, you might see an old, abandoned factory with broken windows that sticks in your mind; this could be your second landmark.

STEP 3 *For every landmark,* mentally place one of the items from your list somewhere beside or in it. So, for the barge you could place the first item on top and, for the factory, you could see the second item in one of the windows. Other landmarks you could use might be monuments, fountains, lampposts, shopwindows, public mailboxes, and so on. The key is to use stationary landmarks that never move, so they will always be there to help you recall your item.

STEP 4 *Continue on your walk,* taking note of your surroundings and placing the items or numbers on your list at key points. At the end of the walk take a moment to breathe. Retrace your steps in your mind, seeing each of the items from your list in place.

STEP 5 *When you repeat the walk the next day,* stay present and aware and take in your surroundings. As you hit each landmark along the way, you should be able to recall each item on your list. Once you have done this a couple of times, you'll find the list of items comes to mind easily just by recalling the walk in your head.

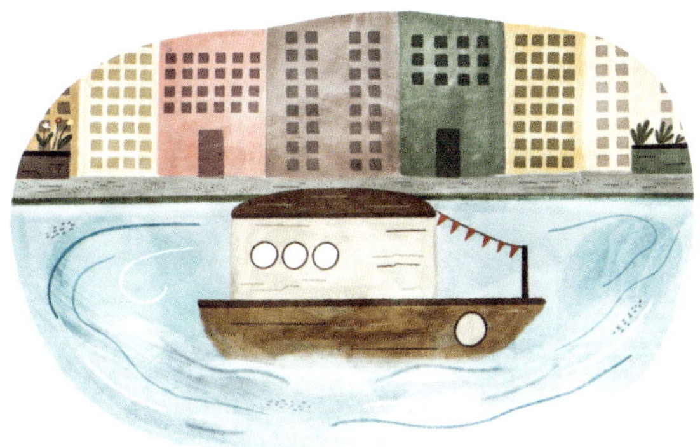

You can do this type of memory exercise with any kind of walk, but a city backdrop provides plenty of material and key locations that you can use as points along the way.

WALK 17

Follow Your Nose

City parks, walkways, and gardens are awash with color for much of the year, but in early spring and summer they really come into their own. As you trail around these open spaces, you'll be greeted with an array of scents, especially if you actively hunt for the aromas. Many borders and hedges are planted with bushy herbs like rosemary, thyme, and lavender, while other astringent beauties, such as sorrel, salvia, and mint, grow in clusters where they can. Then there are the blooms: pretty-in-pink peonies with their sweet, uplifting fragrance combine with climbing roses and scented clematis to add a sugary nuance to the air.

It can be hard to pinpoint exact scents; the real fun lies in identifying the herbs and flowers and appreciating their strength of character and meaning. Even if you don't know the exact name of a plant, it can be an exciting experience to take a fragrant walk through your favorite city park, led purely by the whim of your nose and its preferred scent.

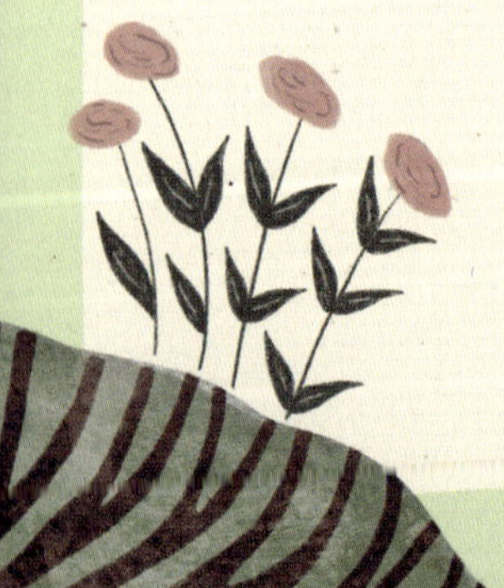

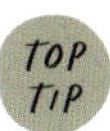

CREATE A FLOWER JOURNAL

Take a notebook with you on your walk and make some notes on your floral finds. Describe them in as much detail as you can, and if you feel inclined, have a go at sketching them. Any details you add will make it easier for you to recall and identify each plant later. Once you've pinpointed your floral discoveries, make a list of the symbolic meanings and folklore associated with each one next to your original notes. It can be great fun to research different blooms and what they represent in mythology, culture, and history. This extra layer of meaning will inevitably add even more enjoyment to your city walks, as you start to recognize and appreciate some of the wildflowers and herbs that grow freely in your patch.

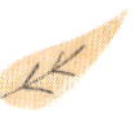

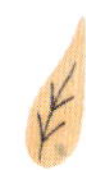

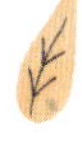

AROMA WALK

An aroma walk is the perfect way to enliven your senses and feel invigorated by your surroundings. The olfactory bulb, where scent signals are processed in the brain, is close to the hippocampus, which is responsible for memory formation. This means that fragrance and emotion are linked. With this in mind, take your time and really connect with each smell. Focus on how the scents make you feel and carry this with you.

- It's a good idea to plan your route before you begin—for example, if you know your local park has lots of wildflowers and herbs, then this would be a good place to start. Alternatively, you might want to take a stroll down a few streets in your neighborhood, taking extra care to pick up on the scents of the flowers and trees as you go.

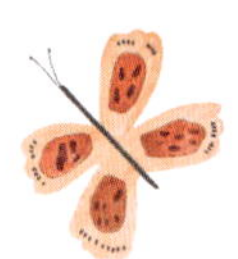

- Limit your walk to forty-five minutes maximum, so you don't suffer olfactory fatigue. If at any point you feel overwhelmed, simply take a few long, deep breaths of fresh air, or sniff the palm of your hand—this acts as a palette cleanser for your nose!
- Relax and check your posture as you walk. Elongate your spine and open your chest by rolling your shoulders back; this will allow you to fully take in the scents as you walk.
- Breathe in deeply through your nose and out slowly through your mouth. This type of walk should be relaxing, so take your time breathing and walking at a comfortable pace.
- Once you have pinpointed a scent that appeals, hold on to it. Follow the source of the fragrance to the flower or plant, so you can appreciate it fully.
- Pay attention not only to what you can smell, but also what you see. Delight in every nuance.
- Try to associate emotions with each fragrance, by asking yourself questions such as "How does this make me feel?" and "What does this remind me of?" Let these thoughts or feelings come to the surface.
- Be tactile during your walk: reach out and gently hold the flower heads to your nose and crush fallen leaves between your fingers to release the scent.
- An aroma walk should be a pleasurable experience, so make it interactive and something that you can reflect upon throughout your day.

WALK 18

Wind Down

The evening brings a different kind of energy to the streets, especially the hours of dusk when the transition from day to night begins. Parks that were once a parade of people and dogs, walking and yapping, slowly quieten as the calmness of the evening draws in. The pathways empty out, apart from a few stragglers and birds picking at the crumbs—remnants of a fun-filled day. The streets are sedate. They experience a lull before the evening's revelers appear. It is an opportunity to breathe and expand, to let the weight of thousands of feet lift from tired slabs. It is time for the early evening walkers to embark on a well-worn path.

THE TURN OF THE SEASONS

The seasons have an influence on each walk you take, but even more so as night draws in. If you're going for a walk in the winter, you will have a very different experience to a dusk ramble in spring or summer. Make the most of this by taking note of the changes and marking them in some way. For example, the crunch of autumn leaves as you wind your way through the park might inspire your poetic side, giving rise to words or even a descriptive chant that you could write down on your return. A spring stroll through the same park might reveal sleepy flower heads, no longer drawn by the sun—capture this by taking a photo on your phone.

A SHAPESHIFTING WALK

If you're the kind of person who needs some time to wind down after a busy day, an early evening walk is the perfect way to do this. Let the charm of the quietening city provide you with the inspiration you need to release the baggage of the day. Watch the changes and learn from them.

- Whether you're walking through the heart of your borough or taking a gentle stroll through the park, you will notice the shift in your surroundings. The way the landscape moves, the dulling of sound, and the dimming of light. The streets become silver rivers at your feet. Every path and walkway looks different as the shadow of darkness descends.

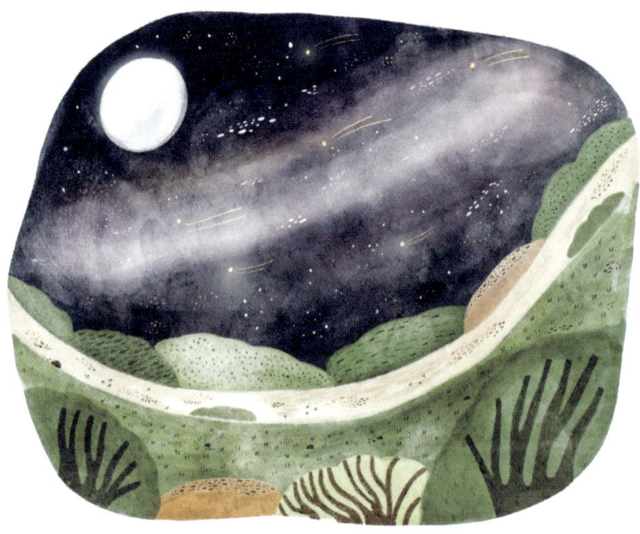

- Where once there was a fusion of color and movement, now there are dark corners peppered with glints of brightness from windows high above. Park railings become black, shiny sentinels, marking the pace of your gait as you walk. The concrete beneath your feet is cold, each dent and crack highlighted in this new vista.

- There's a glimmer of excitement too, for as activity wanes, the sense of something new and magical emerges. Each step along the path takes you farther into the unknown; for while the road is familiar, the flimsy veil of early evening makes everything appear alien.

- As you walk, take a moment to appreciate the changes taking place and feel them within you. Relax your body and mind and go with this. Imagine that with every step the cloak of the day slips further from your shoulders. You can feel it falling, and you're happy to let it go. Like the cityscape, you're shifting shape and becoming something new in order to recharge.

- When you finally feel free of the heaviness of the day, let out a long sigh and appreciate the loss. You might want to pause your walk and spend a minute looking upward at the light of the moon. Imagine the glow, however dim or bright, cloaking you in a sheath of white which cleanses you from head to toe. Continue on your path and be sure to enjoy everything you see, hear, and feel.

WALK 19

Time to Tidy Up

We often walk without thinking about the surroundings we're in or how we have an impact on. City gardens in particular tend to suffer from heavy footfall and the trash left behind by previous pedestrians. Food and pet waste are the key culprits, in addition to cigarette butts, bottle-tops, and paper scraps. While we can't physically reinvent a space that is already established, we can be mindful of our presence, and do our bit to keep things tidy.

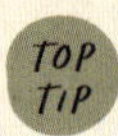

DOING YOUR BIT

If you find litter picking rewarding, you might want to look into local volunteer groups that provide this type of service. You could even start your own group with friends and family in your local community. Urban walking doesn't have to be a solo experience, as walking with others, especially when you have a purpose, can be fun and creates a sense of belonging.

A LITTER-PICKING WALK

Interacting on a small scale helps us stay connected to nature and also adds purpose to a daily stroll. Litter picking is something anyone can do as they walk. It requires little effort, just a keen eye and the motivation to do something for the environment. The rewards are plentiful; you'll improve your focus and gain so much more from the walk. Each little bit you do makes a difference to the space, while reinforcing positive feelings within.

- You will need to take a bag with you and wear protective gloves, as you could be handling any number of items. Be aware of what you pick up and be careful. Avoid glass, sharp objects, and pet waste; instead stick to simple things like paper waste, food wrappers, and plastic.

- You can still enjoy your walk and go at whatever pace suits you; the only difference for this walk is you'll be looking in more detail at your surroundings, so try not to whizz by at such a speed that you miss things. Imagine you're an artist cleaning up a picture.

- Breathe deeply as you walk to energize each step and keep you motivated. Take in the beauty of the park or garden as you go, and feel happy knowing that you are improving this community space by doing your bit.

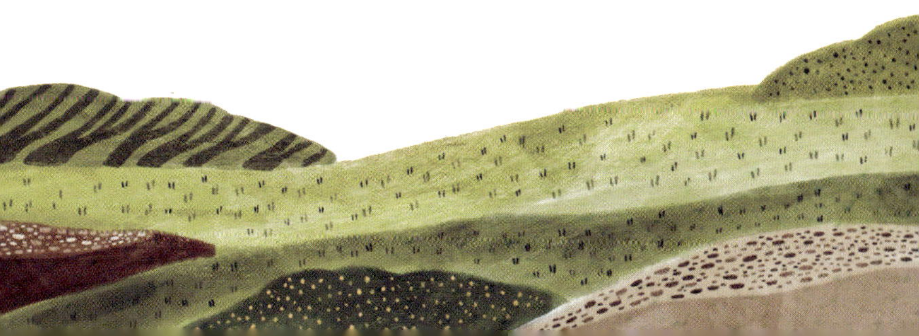

WALK 20

Break Things Up

According to research, taking a short break while doing a walk is as beneficial as the walk itself. It offers a moment of reflection and reinvigorates both body and mind. Resting the body also promotes muscle recovery and allows a short reprieve, which prevents fatigue. Short bursts of vigorous activity also consume more energy overall and burn a higher number of calories.

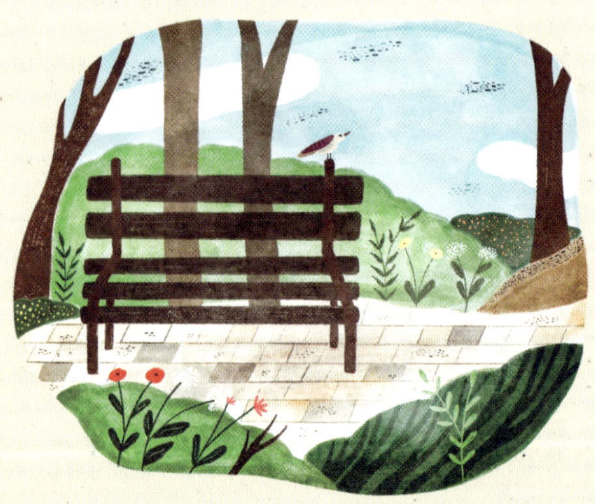

BENCH IT

Make the most of an enforced pause by parking your worries too. During your walk, you may come across a bench or two, from traditional wooden seating to hardy wrought iron or something more contemporary to fit in with a modern urban setting so there are plenty of opportunities to sit and reflect. A wall or even a carefully positioned step are good options too. Once you find somewhere that fits the bill, seize the stillness and take a moment.

STEP 1 *Sit with intent* by placing your bottom firmly on the seat and feeling that connection and support. Allow your shoulders to relax, but open your chest by elongating your spine. Place your feet purposefully on the ground, so you can feel the sidewalk beneath you.

STEP 2 *When you are comfortable,* take a minute to adjust to your surroundings from this position. What do you see, hear, feel, and smell? How do you feel now that you are sitting? You may notice that a particular part of your body is aching, your calf muscles perhaps. Breathe into the pain, and imagine that your breath is soothing it away and energizing each muscle group.

STEP 3 *Reflect upon the walk so far, and how you feel.* Are you enjoying the experience? What have you noticed? If you feel tense or stressed about anything, take this opportunity to park your worries. As you exhale, imagine releasing them into the surrounding space, so when you continue on your route, you leave them behind.

STEP 4 *Give your body a gentle shake* and get moving again. The short break that you have taken should help you feel lighter, brighter, and raring to go!

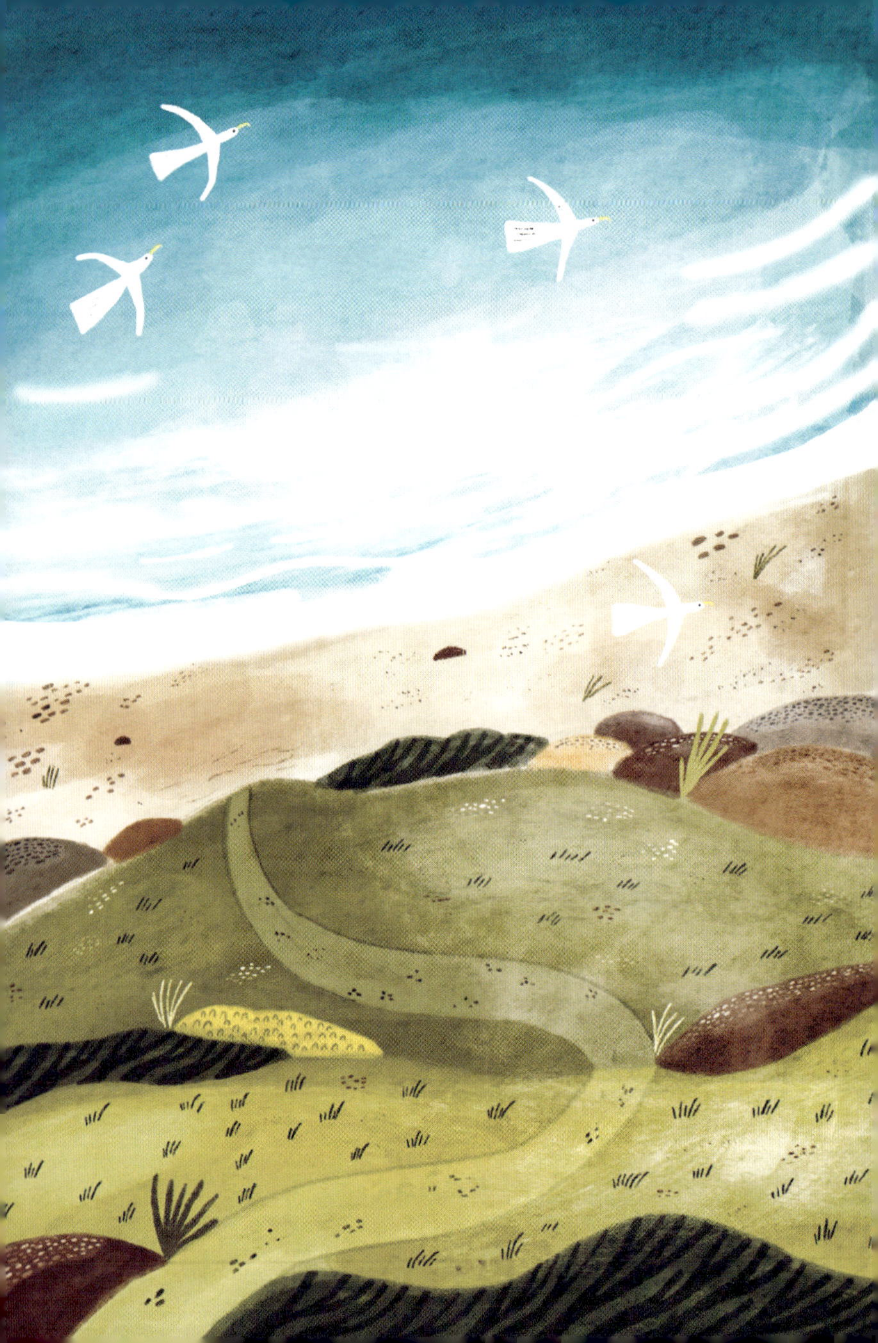

CHAPTER THREE

Seaside Walks

Whether you're looking for a powerfully invigorating walk by the ocean, or a gentle beachside stroll to soothe the soul, you'll find everything you need at the seaside. Walks can be enjoyed at any time of year in this environment, and here you'll find a wealth of mindful and engaging techniques to help you make the most of them.

WALK 21

See the Bigger Picture

Things look different from a great height. A clifftop vista means you'll see and feel more. The distance allows for a much clearer, panoramic viewpoint, so while you're looking at the same beach and shoreline, you can see how far it goes and where it leads. You can also look out toward the horizon and imagine what lies beyond.

The landscape can be rough and jagged underfoot, with sharp slices of rock jutting out, which may make for a challenging walk. However, a coastal cliff walk is rewarding and well worth the extra effort.

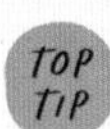

LET GO OF YOUR PROBLEMS

If there is something that is weighing heavy in your life, a problem or stressful situation that you no longer need, use this walk to release it. Carry a small shell, feather, or flower with you and when you reach the point where you pause and take in the view, use this moment to let it go. Take a long, deep breath in and, as you exhale, hold the item in both hands and imagine pouring all your worries into it. Cast the item over the cliff edge and say, "I release you." Then continue on your path, feeling lighter and brighter.

CLIFFTOP TREK

Use a clifftop walk as an opportunity to broaden your horizons and find some peace. Use the view as a meditation prompt, to help you zone out and find a moment of stillness and clarity. The following tips to help you get the most from your walk:

- Make sure you're kitted out in appropriate clothing for a cliff hike. You'll need plenty of layers, including a windproof and waterproof outer layer, as the weather can change quickly on the coast. Good, sturdy walking boots with a deep tread will help you navigate a rocky terrain. Walking poles can also help you maintain balance. Ensure you have water, energy snacks, a fully charged phone, and navigational tools like a compass or map.

- Check the weather report before you leave home. Avoid high winds when you're taking a clifftop amble and be sure to walk along the designated path. It might seem tempting to deviate or get closer to the edge for the view, but always put your safety first.

- Notice the direction of the wind. Can you feel it whipping around your legs? Is it pushing you forward, carrying the weight of each step and encouraging you on your journey? Perhaps you're facing into the wind and you can feel the resistance of the breeze against your body. Press into this and notice how the air supports you. Breathe deeply and recognize how the same air fills your lungs and clears your head. Feel the breeze as it brushes against your face and through your hair.

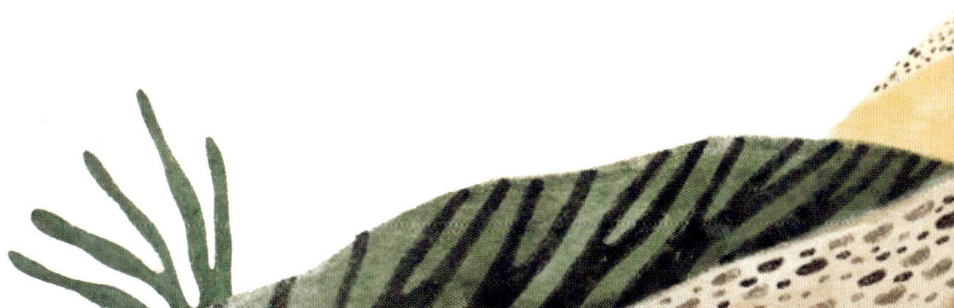

- Look at the view directly ahead of you. What can you see in your eyeline? Perhaps you can see the sweeping landscape, the tips of craggy rocks in the distance, and the undulating line of the land. Look out to sea and follow the shoreline with your eyes. See the point where the sky meets the sea and notice the change in color and movement. Pause and take a moment to drink in the view. How does it make you feel? The vast canvas of the sea is eternal as it stretches out before you. You may feel small against the infinite swathe of coast Imagine what is beyond the horizon. Think about the possibilities and opportunities that lie ahead. Focus solely on the emptiness, on the line between limitless air and the fluid, flowing water of the sea. Breathe, relax, and let this stillness consume you.

- Take steady steps and deep breaths and take note of everything you see—the birds soaring in the sky, the people on the beach below, the frothy waves that roll toward the shore; take it all in. Know that with every step your head will become clearer, your heart lighter, and your focus sharper.

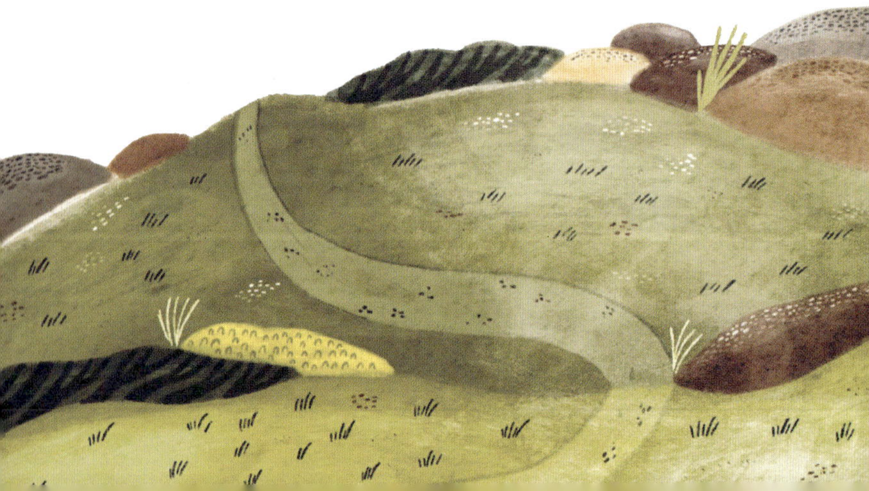

WALK 22

Make Your Mark

If you crave the feeling of sand between your toes, there's a reason—it's naturally good for you! Sand has shock-absorbing properties which cushion each footfall. This means it's much gentler on the joints, making it excellent for those who suffer with arthritis. Navigating the uneven terrain barefoot also helps to redistribute body weight, allowing for a more natural foot motion that strengthens the ankle muscles. Research suggests that it may also improve the immune system, thanks to the direct flow of electrons from the Earth into the body, which has an antioxidant effect.

The softness of the sand is nurturing and it's thought that this natural contact stimulates the vagus nerve, an important part of the nervous system that regulates emotional response and promotes relaxation. Couple this with the calming effect of being close to water, and you have the perfect antidote to everyday stress.

SANDY SUMMER STROLL

Use a relaxing beach walk on a sunny day as an opportunity to rebalance body and mind and engage with the elements of Air, Water, Fire, and Earth. Use the time to reflect upon your journey in the present moment.

STEP 1 *Find a stretch of sandy beach that is safe to walk on barefoot, and take off your shoes*. Choose a pleasant day when the sun is out and it's not too chilly, so you can relax and enjoy the experience fully. If possible, begin your walk close to the sea where the sand is moist and you can see and hear the waves lapping upon the shore.

STEP 2 *As you walk, allow your feet to roll forward comfortably from heel to toe*, so they make an impression in the damp sand. Notice the sound of the sand as it envelops your feet. Feel the wet, grainy softness against your skin and let it squeeze up through your toes to fully engulf each foot. It might feel strange at first, but try to relax and go with the sensation; you'll soon get used to it.

STEP 3 *Let the elements embrace you.* Breathe deeply and let the sound of the sea relax you. Taste the salty breeze upon the tip of your tongue and notice how it awakens your entire mouth. Notice too how the air infuses you with energy and propels you forward on your walk. The rolling waves rush to greet you; the trickling sound as water seeps into sand is comforting and the movement spurs you onward. The heat of the sun, a fiery ball of energy in the sky, warms your skin and the light makes the sandy vista sparkle with a brightness that cheers you. Notice how the warmth and the sunlight lift your mood.

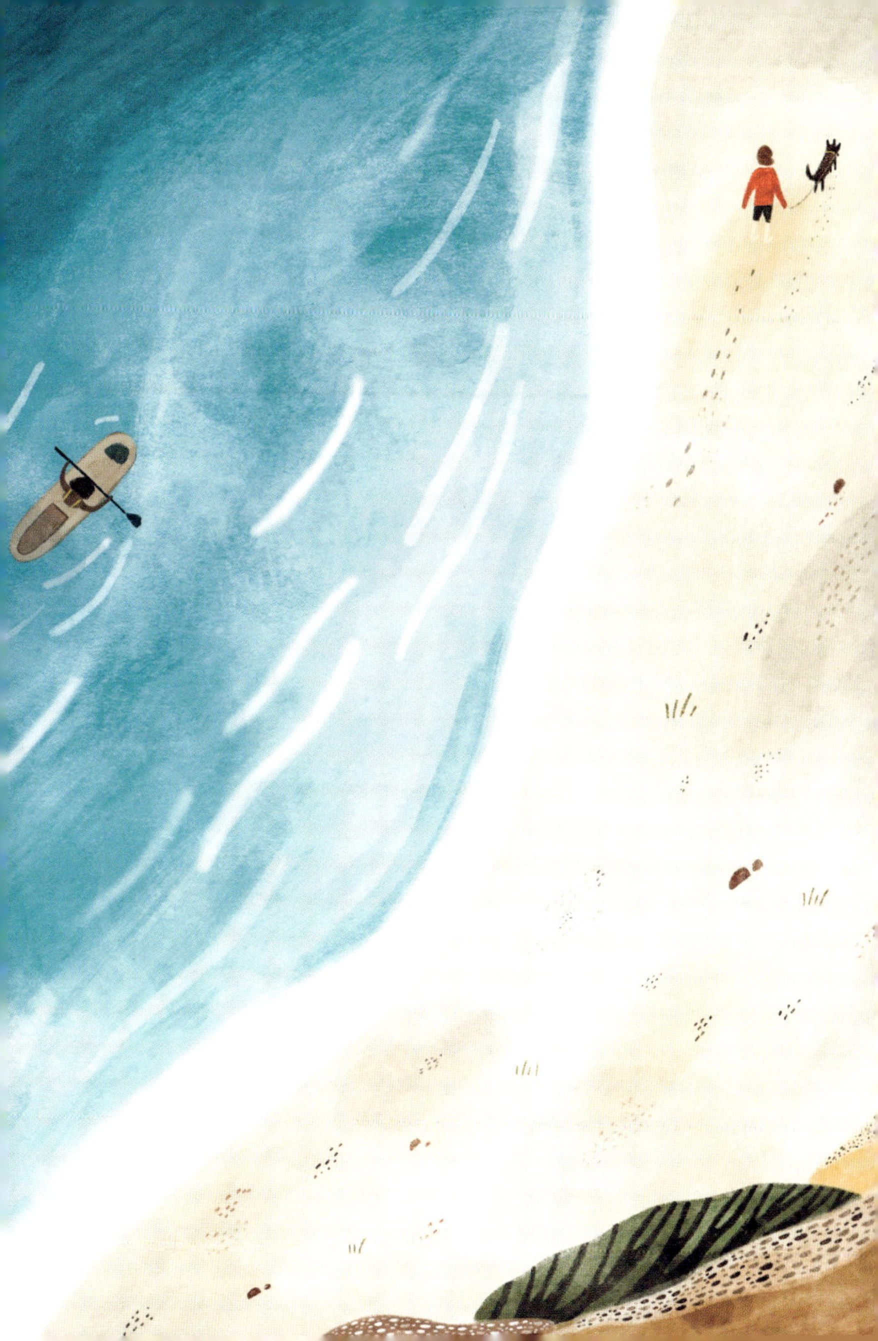

STEP 4 *Close your eyes for a few seconds as you walk, and notice what you feel in your body.* Perhaps the wet sand clinging to your feet holds your attention: the way it gives each step extra bounce and helps you feel grounded. It could be the breeze buffeting your body and tugging at your hair, or perhaps it's the smell, the scent of sea and seaweed, of salt and brine.

STEP 5 *Cast an eye over your shoulder and look at the footprints you have left in the sand,* a transient reminder of where you've been and how far you have come. Some may have already been stolen by the tide, but that doesn't matter because you know the steps you have taken to get to this point. You are fully aware and present for this journey.

STEP 6 *Begin to walk farther inland,* where the sand is dry, and notice how this shift in landscape feels. It's a different kind of softness, a powdery coarseness that exfoliates your skin gently as you stroll. Relax and sink your feet deep into the earth. Know that thousands of people have passed the same way, and that you are walking in their footsteps.

WALK 23

Promenade with Your Pup

Taking a dog walk by the sea benefits both owner and pet. The range of sights, sounds, and smells provide mental stimulation and the wide-open space is the perfect playground for excitable dogs to get plenty of exercise and have some fun. Many dogs love to paddle or swim, as the cool water helps to regulate their temperature on a hot summer's day, and it's a sensory experience. There's the opportunity for social interaction with other dogs, and a walk together is a bonding experience, which strengthens the ties between human and dog. It's also a great way for owners to get their daily dose of exercise.

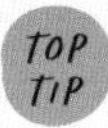

BRING A BOTTLE

The beach might be surrounded by water, but it's important for you and your dog to stay hydrated, so bring plenty of fresh drinking water with you. Encourage your dog to take regular breaks, especially if it's a longer walk in the heat, so you can both have a drink and a snack. Be aware of the weather. If it's a baking hot day, do this walk either early in the morning or later in the evening.

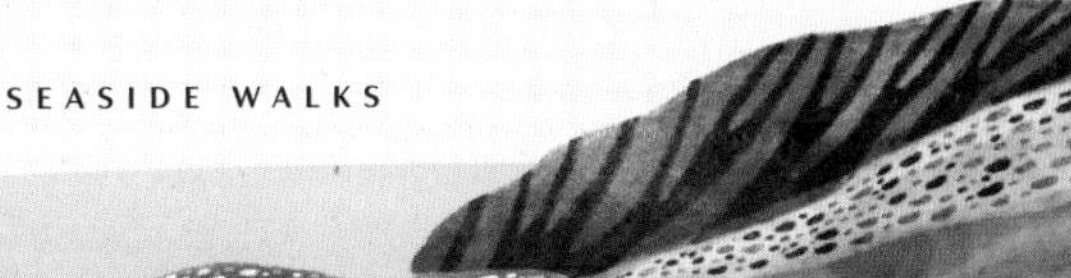

BEACH DOG WALK

Let your dog inspire you, as you walk along the shoreline. Watch how they act and engage with their surroundings and then follow their lead. Connect with your playful inner child and experience the beach through your dog's eyes.

- While you might usually use a leash to take your dog for a walk, get into some role reversal and let your dog take the lead in a beach adventure. Allow them to set the pace, and go where their nose takes you. If the beach is busy, you might have to put your dog on a leash, but, if possible, go early so they can run free.

- Appreciate your dog's sense of fun and watch what they're doing. Notice how their inquisitive nature takes over once they're given free rein.

- Get into the playful spirit and join your dog for a frolic by the water's edge. Let your dog's enthusiasm rub off on you by diving straight in. Plunge your bare feet into the water without hesitation and enjoy the refreshing rush of energy that you feel as you do this. Splash around and make some noise: remember what it was like as a child running through the sea and engage with that feeling.

- If your dog is sprinting ahead, match their pace with a brisk walk. Take long, purposeful strides to catch them up and notice how this changes your breathing pattern.

- When your dog pauses to check something out, take a minute to rest and soak in your surroundings.

- Notice what you can smell: are there any interesting aromas in the air?
- Notice too what you can see: do a slow spin around and get the full panoramic view.
- Notice what you can feel: perhaps you can feel the sand between your toes or your dog brushing against you. Enjoy these feelings of closeness.
- If your dog has found something interesting on the beach, check it out with them. If it's a piece of driftwood, you can use it as a toy to throw. Be inventive and create new games that you can play together using your beach finds.

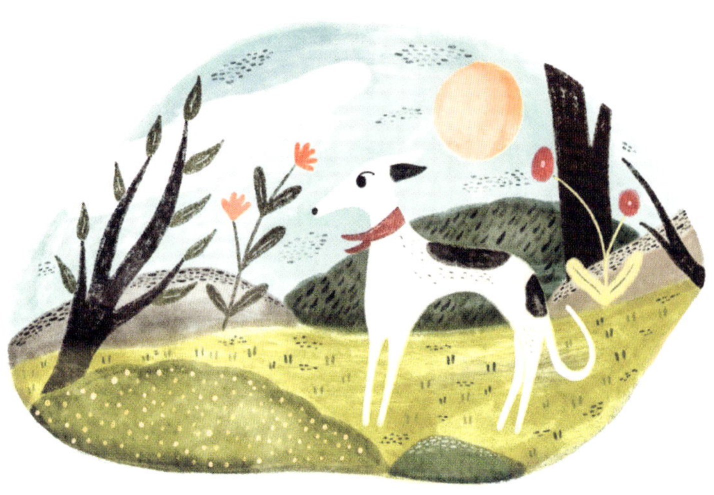

WALK 24

Wade in the Water

Seawater is good for you! It has many properties that can be absorbed through the skin—which makes a paddle in the waves a reviving and therapeutic experience. The sea is rich in minerals like magnesium, calcium, and iodine, which can benefit thyroid function and bone health, while the salty sea air, which is more potent along the shoreline, helps to clear the airways and reduce respiratory inflammation. The deeper you wade, the more you'll benefit, as the resistance of the water also helps to tone and strengthen muscles.

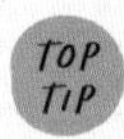

MAKE TIME TO PLAY

Take a break from your walk for some creative fun. Find a patch of sand and draw a pattern in it with your toes, or have a go at writing your name. If you prefer, take a moment to sit down and build a sandcastle. A playful rest will rejuvenate your spirit and also give you the energy and motivation to finish your walk.

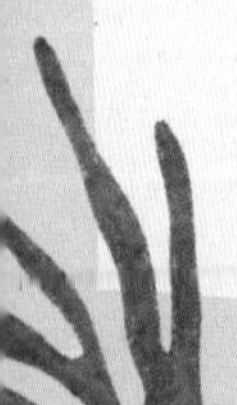

MOOD-BOOSTING WALK

The seaside often summons childhood memories, bringing to mind carefree times and positive emotions. This type of vista is ideal if you're looking for a walk to lift your mood. Engage your senses and let your playful side emerge as you stroll along the shoreline.

STEP 1 *Take off your shoes and socks,* roll up your pants legs, and prepare to have some fun!

STEP 2 *Paddle along the edge of the water where the sand is wet,* so you can experience the intermittent waves as they lap against the shore. Try not to brace yourself as the cool water hits; instead, open up and embrace the sudden impact.

STEP 3 *Each time a wave comes,* take a deep, exhilarating breath and then exhale and release any pent-up tension. Imagine it being washed away by the retreating water.

STEP 4 *If you feel brave enough, go in deeper,* so the sea comes up to your ankles. You might feel a slight resistance the deeper you go, as the sea clings to your skin and the tide does its own thing. It doesn't matter; you have the power to carve a path through the waves and reach your destination.

STEP 5 *Pick up your pace now and enjoy the moment.* Jump, skip, and splash, and recall what it was like as a child to run through water, to paddle along the shore. Remember how the sensation of water and sand made you feel, and go back to that in your mind. Allow your innate playfulness to rise to the surface.

WALK 25

Be More Scavenger

Throughout history humans have foraged along the coastline. Early civilizations relied upon the sea as a method of transport and a key food source; they spent thousands of years scavenging beaches and saltmarshes for sustenance. The variety of coastal habitats, including craggy sea cliffs, sandy dunes, tide pools at low tide, and also mudflats and estuaries, offers the potential for a range of finds.

Whether you're looking for an edible feast, or seeking out shoreline treasures that can be used in crafting or as mementos to decorate your home, you'll find everything you need on a seaside walk.

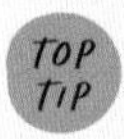

DO YOUR RESEARCH

Know what you're looking for and where to find it. Seaweeds like rockweed, kelp, and dulse are edible and found along rocky beaches. You may also find dewberries and wild leeks in or around sand dunes. Check out holes in the sand for clams. Mussels and sea snails can also be foraged at low tide. You'll find an array of decorative finds along the beach, including sea glass, shells, pebbles, driftwood, and even fossils.

TREASURE-HUNTING WALK

To scavenge, you need an open mind and the ability to see beyond the surface. It helps if you know what you're looking for, and you need to be prepared to dig deep and look beneath the detritus to identify a real find. Whether you're after tasty morsels to eat or something unique as a keepsake like a pretty shell or stone, a foraging walk will sharpen your focus and stimulate your innate creativity.

- Preparation is key, so before you go on your walk, check for low tide timings; consult a reputable tide chart and make sure you won't be cut off at any point if the tide starts to come in. Be selective when it comes to the stretch of coastline you'll be foraging. Avoid areas close to industrial sites and check for pollution. Also make sure you keep away from areas that have algal blooms, as this makes any edible finds toxic.

- Have the right equipment with you. Wear waterproof shoes and protective gloves, so you can handle your finds safely. Take a waterproof flashlight, so you can see into tide pools and crevices. You'll need bags to keep your foraged finds in.

- You can go at any pace on this type of walk, but you want to spot as much as possible, so don't rush.

- Scour the ground as you go and have an idea of what you're hoping to find, as this will dictate the direction of your walk. For example, if you're looking for seaweed, you'll need to look higher along the beach, but if you're hoping to find sea beet or samphire, you'll have to probe between rocks and in among the sand dunes.

- Be respectful as you walk. Replace rocks and stones that you've lifted and only take what you need. Drink in the atmosphere and give thanks for the gifts of the sea.

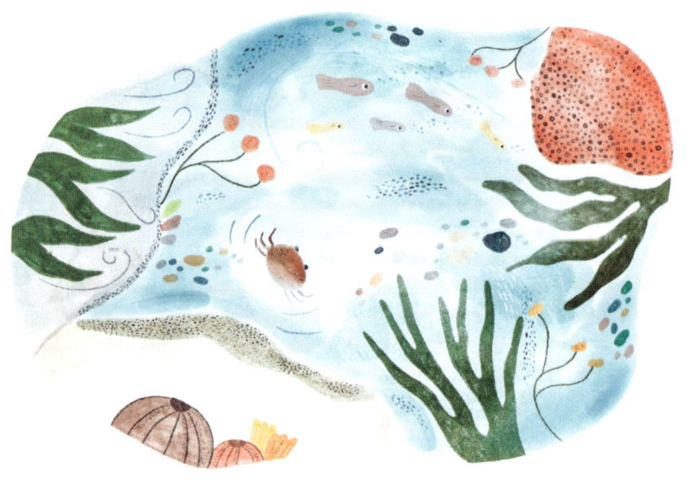

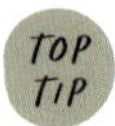

KEEP A JOURNAL

This type of trek helps you reconnect with the natural world and your ancestors, as you're following the old ways and walking a path that they would have taken. When you reach the end of your beach walk, reflect upon the journey in a journal. Use the following questions as prompts:

- *What did you enjoy about it?*
- *What, if anything, did you find uncomfortable?*
- *How does it feel to know that you have walked the same path as thousands of others?*
- *Consider the path you walk in life, and how your ancestors paved the way for you.*
- *Consider too the journey you have taken so far, and how far you have come. How does this make you feel?*

Embrace the Chill

The winter casts a very different light on the shoreline. Frost-tipped sand dunes glimmer under the low sunlight, while the air is tinged with an icy chill. Waves thunder and roll, whipped up into a frenzy by the bracing wind. They crash against the cliffs, the salty spray adding a dense richness to the slick gray stone. There's an emptiness to this picture, a space waiting to be filled. Beaches are secluded, the choppy sea left to its own devices, but that doesn't mean there is nothing of interest to see. This is the perfect time to appreciate the landscape and spot wildlife doing its own thing.

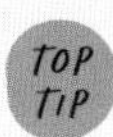

EXPLORE THE LANDSCAPE

Explore the craggy coastline as you walk. You might notice caves or alcoves in the cliffs. If so, take a minute to appreciate these natural wonders. Reach out and touch the stone, peek inside, and see what you can find. Gaze into tide pools and look for signs of life. Imagine you're an explorer who has come to this land for the first time. What would you think? What would pique your interest? Look with fresh eyes and enjoy the landscape.

WINDY WINTER WALK

Cooler weather clears the head and provides an opportunity to find peace. All you have to do is be open and let your senses take the lead. Embrace the drop in temperature and let the wind work its cleansing magic. A winter walk along the coastline helps you reconnect with the natural world.

- Be mindful of the weather and don't venture out if it's too windy or during a thunderstorm.
- Wrap up warm. It's always colder by the coast, so you'll need lots of layers and waterproofs. A thermal hat, scarf, and gloves are key accessories.
- Steer clear of clifftops in case the wind picks up. Instead, opt for a beach stroll, but be aware that the sand can sometimes be slippery underfoot.
- As you walk, observe the vista. Notice how different it looks during the winter months.
- Take note of the light and the color of the sand and notice how the sea takes on a smoky, silvery hue.
- Feel the difference in temperature, the icy chill of the breeze upon your cheeks, and the way it pushes against your body as you walk.
- Put extra effort into each step, press into the resistance of the wind, and let it support you.
- Take longer, deeper breaths to infuse you with energy. Feel the cool air settle in your lungs and hold it there. Release each breath through pursed lips.

- Let the flow of the tide spur you onward.
- Look out to the horizon and draw in the emptiness, the space, and the potential in that view.
- Look down at your feet: what can you see?
- You may spot a stick or a slender piece of driftwood. If so, pick it up and use it to create art by drawing and doodling patterns in the sand as you stroll.
- Place all your attention on what you are doing, whether you're walking, looking out to sea, or making patterns in the sand. If worries or stresses come into your mind, simply acknowledge them and then let them go. Imagine the power of the wind carrying them away.
- Enjoy the beauty and serenity of a secluded beach. Let it soothe your soul as you continue to walk.

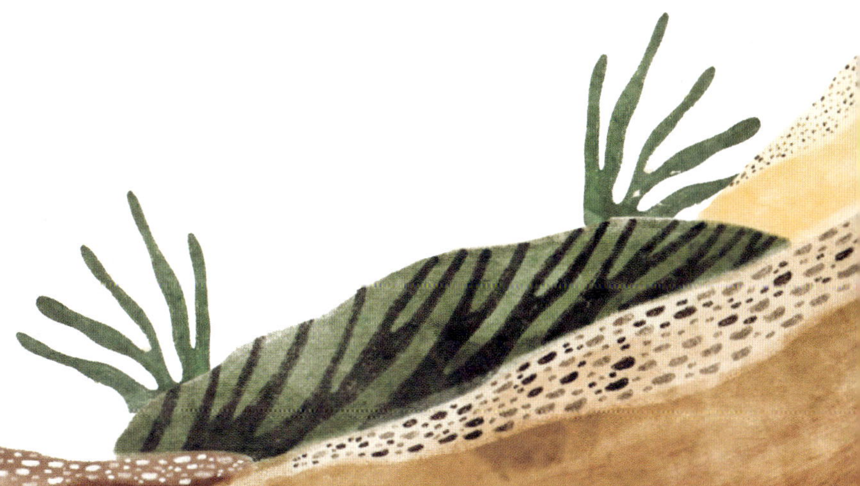

WALK 27

Celebrate the Sun

There is nothing more captivating than a beach sunrise. This beautiful breathtaking sight promotes a positive mindset for the rest of the day, but it has other benefits too. The early morning burst of vitamin D boosts health, while the sunlight resets the body's circadian rhythm. This regulates snoozing patterns and contributes to a restful night's sleep. According to research, the feeling of awe that is experienced while watching a sunrise has an anti-inflammatory effect on the body, improving the immune system, while the light absorbed by the retinas in each eye triggers the brain to produce serotonin, the feel-good chemical that lifts the mood.

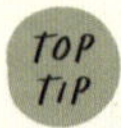

ENJOY A BEACH PICNIC

Take a simple picnic with you and enjoy a beach breakfast. You don't want to be weighed down, so choose something light like a couple of pieces of fruit and some water. Find a spot along the shoreline where you can sit in comfort and take in the beauty of the sunrise. Use this time to recharge and set your intentions for the day ahead.

SUNRISE WALK

Set your alarm early, so that you can catch the sunrise as you walk along the beach. Use this quiet time to reset your thoughts and generate positive energy. All you need to do is, relax, absorb the golden rays, and let the beach setting inspire you

The key is to take your time with this walk, treat it as your waking up time, and let your body and mind gently adjust to the day ahead.

To reap the most benefits, choose a long stretch of sandy beach, so you can walk barefoot. The connection that you feel to the earth will help to anchor you and stimulate your senses. You'll have to put more effort in while walking on a sandy surface and over the course of the walk you can build up pace to boost energy levels.

STEP 1 *Start walking when it is still dark*, so you can watch the sunrise unfold. Notice the first chinks of light on the horizon, and appreciate the gentle glow that emanates along the skyline and how it gradually brightens as the sun comes up.

STEP 2 *Breathe with purpose and intention*; inhale deeply and imagine that with every breath you're turning up the brightness of your own aura. This is the energy field that surrounds the body. Picture it as a cloak of light surrounding you. See it changing color like the sky, absorbing the rose-pink light that burns brightly on the horizon. Feel it transforming into a deep golden red and then burning with a vibrant, orange-yellow shimmer.

STEP 3 *Feel the warmth of the sun's rays upon your skin* as you take each step. Imagine the sun spurring you onward, awakening your body and mind. Notice how it eases aching muscles and gives you the strength to move forward.

STEP 4 *Elongate your spine as you walk and lift your head to the sun*. Stride forward, increasing your pace, and greet the day with a wide smile upon your face. Say an affirmation to put you in a positive mindset, something like, "I rise like the sun and let my light shine!" Enjoy this feeling of renewal as you continue your walk.

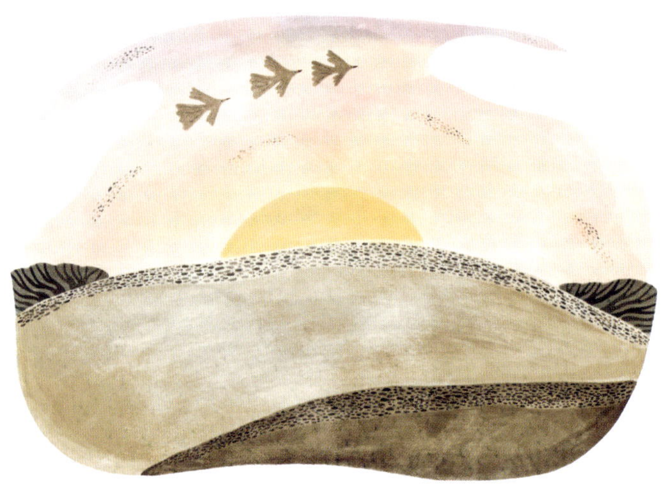

WALK 28

Look at the Stars

Coastal stargazing is a popular pastime, and a great way to enhance an evening beach walk. The wide-open space and reduced light pollution provide a perfect starry canvas, so, if you're a beginner, you'll find it much easier to locate constellations with the naked eye.

When the moon is low in the sky, there's a chance you'll see the 'glitter path' forming. This glimmering line of light is created by the moon's reflection in the surface of the water. While you're looking up, be sure to look out to sea too, as you may spot bioluminescent plankton in the waves.

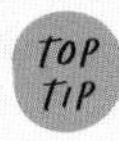

PREPARATION IS KEY

Before you go on your walk, have an idea of what you'd like to see. Find out which planets are visible at the time you are venturing out, and also check out any constellations you might see. Keep an eye on news reports in case there's anything unusual going on in the sky—for example, meteor showers or the opportunity to see the Northern Lights. There are some great stargazing apps, which can help you locate interesting objects in the night sky, so keep your phone handy.

RELAXING STARGAZING STROLL

Give your eyes a treat by combining an evening walk along the beach with some stargazing. The beach setting, together with the beauty of the night sky, is awe-inspiring and promotes deep relaxation, which will help you have a restful sleep.

STEP 1 *Wait for dusk*, as the sun is slowly setting in the sky, and take an evening stroll along the beach. Wrap up warm as there may well be a sudden dip in temperature as night draws in.

STEP 2 *As you walk, take in the changing light*, and watch as the colors of the sky transform before your eyes. Notice the vibrant pinks and the soft orange glow as the sunlight dwindles. Breathe deeply and let this gentle shift to warming hues soothe your soul.

STEP 3 *When the sun is finally swallowed by darkness, take the opportunity to stop and gaze upward.* Look at the blanket of sky above you and lose yourself in the pattern of the stars.

STEP 4 *See if you can find the North Star (Polaris) or Canopus*, some of the brightest in the sky, and pick out any constellations. If you don't recognize any of these, simply enjoy the spectacle as it unfolds. Let your imagination do the work and come up with patterns, images, and symbols in the stars.

STEP 5 *Gaze at the moon as you walk*, noticing its shape and size and the soft shimmering glow that it casts upon the sea. Breathe in and imagine you are bathed from head to toe in moonlight.

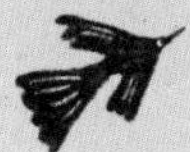

THINGS TO LOOK OUT FOR:

The seaside often summons childhood memories, bringing to mind carefree times and positive emotions. This type of vista is ideal if you're looking for a walk to lift your mood. Engage your senses, and let your playful side emerge as you stroll along the shoreline.

Planets
These look like bright stars, but they don't twinkle. Some planets are tinged with color. Mars, for example, has a reddish hue, while Jupiter is pale yellow in shade. Planets are most visible in clear coastal skies just after sunset during the winter months, when the sky is dark and clear.

Comets
These are bright balls of dust and ice heated by the sun, with a tail trailing off into the distance. They appear hazy to the naked eye due to the gases surrounding the nucleus.

Zodiacal Light
This eerie glow, which emanates upward from the horizon and can often be cone-shaped, is caused by sunlight reflected by cometary dust in the Solar System, particularly on the ecliptic plane. It's visible in dark, clear skies, usually just after sunset or before sunrise.

Meteor Showers
These bright streaks of light, sometimes called shooting stars, seem to appear from nowhere. They have a tapered tail that fades toward the end.

Star Clusters
If you have binoculars, you might be able to spot star clusters, or nebulae, in the distance. These glowing clouds of dust and gas are usually visible against a dark horizon and illuminated by nearby stars.

WALK 29

See the Seashells

You might think that seashells are just pretty beach adornments, but they are also the home of the mollusks, a group of soft-bodied invertebrate, which includes snails, periwinkles, clams, mussels, oysters, and slugs. The seashell that you find on a beach stroll is a carefully crafted exoskeleton made from proteins and calcium carbonate. It grows gradually with the mollusk, getting bigger as the creature ages. While it's hard to pinpoint the exact number of shells in the world, estimates suggest that there could be anything from 50,000 to 200,000 different species, so there are lots of different types to discover on a seaside walk.

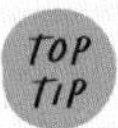

CREATE BEACH ART

Use your finds to trigger your artistic side. It's up to you how you do this. You might choose your favorite shell and have a go at sketching it, there and then on the sand, or in the comfort of your own home. If you prefer, take a small handful of your favorites with you, clean them up, and create a shell collage, or arrange them in a decorative dish that you can place in your bathroom. This will remind you of the sea and your walk, as you relax in the bath to recharge and set your intentions for the day ahead.

SHELL-SEEKING WALK

The beach is the ideal environment to hone your observation skills. It's a wide-open space, which makes it easier for you to explore and find what you're looking for, especially if you sharpen your focus and concentrate on your feet as you stroll.

The aim of this walk is to stay present and filter out external noise by concentrating on one thing. You're going to make shells your primary target and the idea is to collect a range that appeal to you as you walk along the shore.

- You will need a bag of some description to put your finds in. Keep your phone handy too, as this will help you identify the different types.
- You'll need to find a long stretch of beach and begin your walk along the beach drift where the sea has left most of the shells. This is higher up the shoreline where the sand is dry.
- Make sure you attempt this exercise at low tide, as more of the beach will be exposed and you'll be able to find recently deposited shells.
- Also consider the time of day. If possible, go early in the morning, especially if this aligns with a lower tide, as the beach is likely to be quieter, which means you'll be able to cover more ground.
- A shell-seeking walk is a lot of fun, especially if you're in a group with family or friends. You'll be able to compare finds and you are more likely to discover something interesting, with more pairs of eyes on the case.

- Take your time and enjoy the walk. Scour the sand in a sweeping motion. Look out for bright colors, spikes, and patterns that catch your eye. Focus solely on the land and what you can see.

- Pause and inspect your finds: this isn't a walk that you can rush. Consider yourself a shell detective, searching for clues.

- Tide pools are an excellent place to look for shells, so if you see any along your walk, take the time to peer in. Use this moment as an opportunity for a moment of stillness. Place all your attention solely on the tide pool, breathe deeply, and remain motionless, and you will be more likely to spot something of interest.

- If you do find a shell, be careful that there isn't a creature living inside. You may also find tiny fish and crabs.

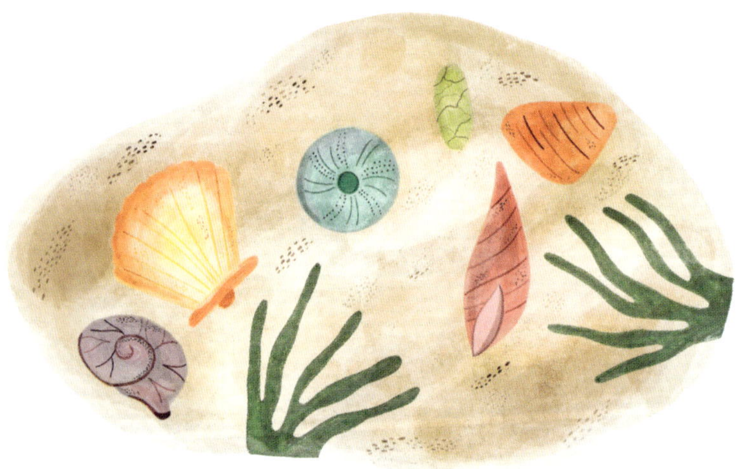

THINGS TO LOOK OUT FOR:

The swell of the sand dunes and damper tidal stretches offer an opportunity to sharpen your observation skills. The gleaming jeweled shells and pallid pretties that lay hidden at your feet are easier to spot when you know what you're looking for. Pay attention as you walk and you'll be rewarded with some memorable finds. Items to look out for include:

Single-shelled mollusks like conchs, whelks, and cowries. Conch shells are usually large and spiral-shaped with a flared lip; whelks are similar in shape but are often more elongated; while cowries look almost jewel-like with their small, rounded, and glossy appearance.

Clams are easy to spot. These mollusks are oval or round, and have two halves which are connected by an adjoining valve.

Scallops are a decorative find. These textured, fan-shaped shells come in a variety of colors, from red and orange to purple, yellow, and white.

Mussels are bivalves, like clams and scallops, meaning they are comprised of two interconnected shells. They are roughly oblong in shape and usually deep blue to purple in hue.

Winkles or periwinkles are conical and whorled, often patterned with lines and usually black, gray, or dark brown.

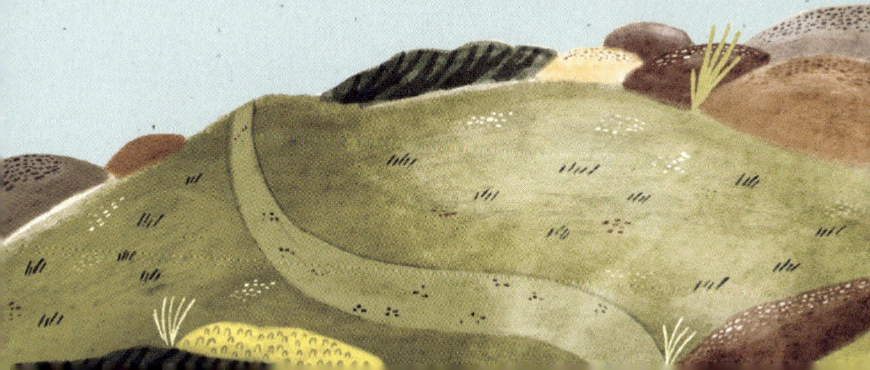

WALK 30

Let the Sounds of the Sea Soothe You

Research shows that listening to the gentle, rhythmic music of the ocean causes an increase in the production of neurochemicals like dopamine and oxytocin, which elevate the mood and reduce anxiety. The low-frequency noise of the sea also has a soothing effect on the body. The sound of rolling waves triggers the parasympathetic nervous system, which helps to reduce stress and induce a sense of calm, while also lowering blood pressure.

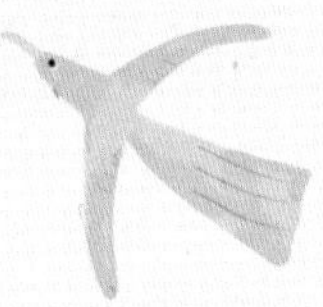

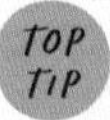

A SOUNDSCAPE ON REPEAT

When you have finished your walk, continue the idea of a creating a theme tune throughout your day, or whenever you need a moment of calm. Wherever you are walking, you can recreate the sounds of the sea in your mind by visualizing the setting and recalling its soothing symphony. Hear the waves crashing against the shore, hear their steady rhythm, and let the sound take you on a journey back to the coast. Let your body flow in time with the music in your head and reconnect with those peaceful feelings.

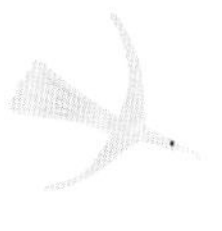
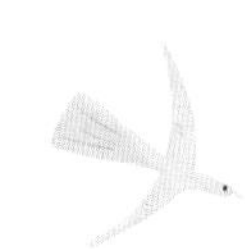

SOUND STROLLING

Whether you're following the shoreline, a stony coastline, or walking with the ocean in the distance, let the sounds of the sea accompany your journey. Focus on the rhythmic lilt of the waves to balance the emotions and promote peace.

- As you walk, train your focus, so while you might hear the noise of traffic in the distance or people on the beach talking, you block this out by concentrating solely on the sound of the waves as they surge toward the shore. Every time your attention wanes or you find yourself pulled away by other sounds, return to the waves.

- It can help if you time your breathing to match the tidal flow, so make the in and out motion of the waves your prompt for every inward and outward breath.

- Notice layers of sound as you walk. For example, if you're close to the shoreline, you might hear the rush of the water as it runs up the beach. You might hear the wind whistling upon the surface of the sea or birds overhead. Where do these sounds fall in the rhythmic motion of the waves? How do they fit into the ocean's overture?

- Let this soothing music be your theme tune, and move in time with it. Make each step fluid and appreciate the flexibility of your body as you walk.

- Imagine the waves washing over you as you walk, cleansing you fully and removing any negative thoughts or feelings as they ebb and flow.

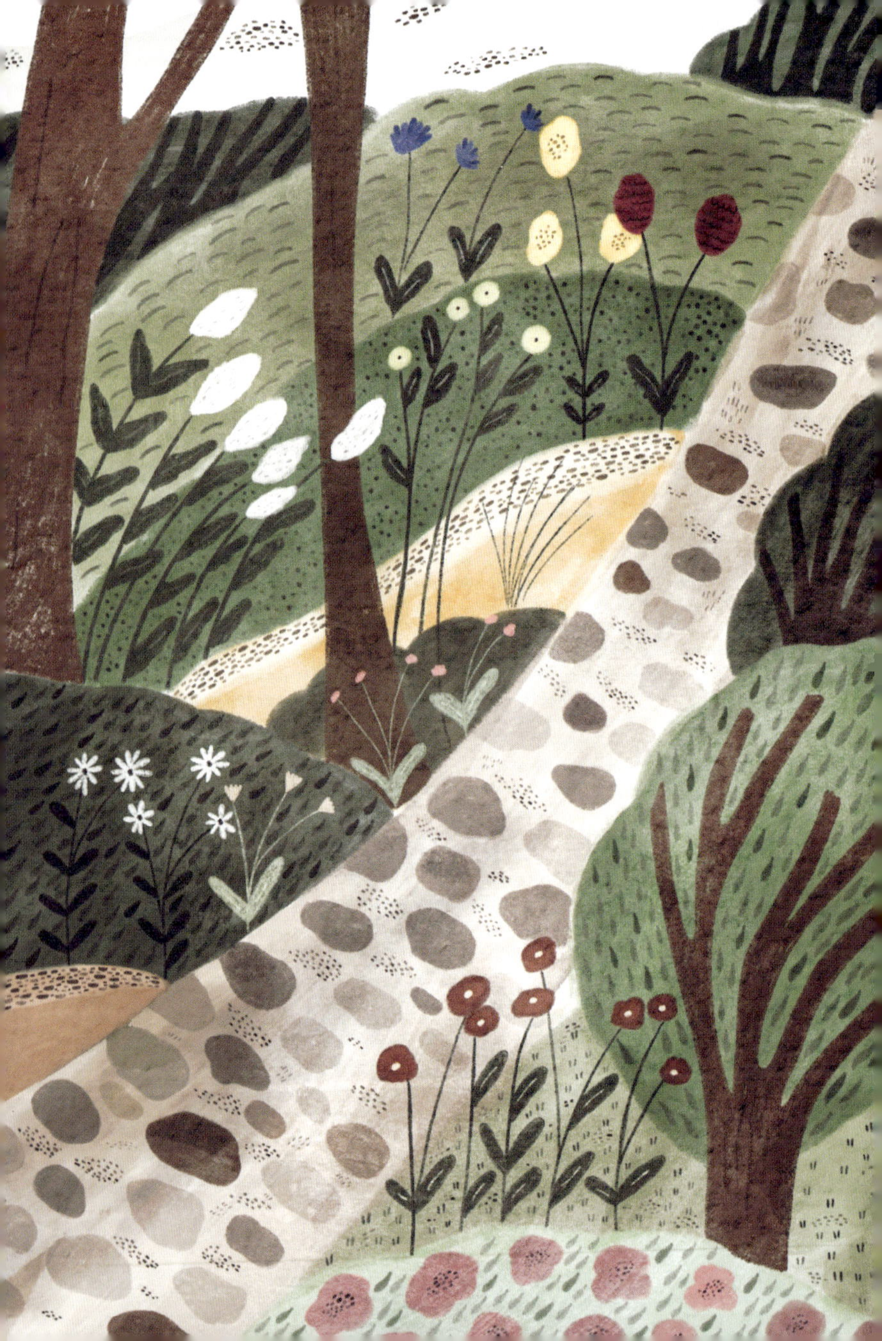

CHAPTER FOUR

Short Strolls

A short walk replenishes the brain, and it also boosts attention levels, alleviates stress, and lifts the mood, according to scientific research. The fresh air, regular exercise, and social interaction, especially if you're walking with a friend, helps you feel more energized and increases self-esteem. What's not to love?

WALK 31

Go Off the Beaten Track

A short stroll doesn't have to be boring. While there are many benefits to taking a well-worn route, especially if time is limited, you can mix things up by going off the beaten track. If something piques your interest, take it a step further. Stimulate your innate curiosity and peek down that lane that always catches your eye, or turn left when you would normally go right. You'll find out where the path leads and may even discover a secret garden or tree-lined track that adds a little extra magic to your day.

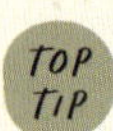

TURN THINGS AROUND

Sometimes taking the opposite direction to your normal route will open up a world of new experiences. With this in mind, choose your favorite short walk and flip it on its head by doing it in reverse. Enter the park at the gate you would normally leave by, turn right around the pond instead of left, and so on. This might feel strange at first, but you'll be amazed at the difference it makes. Once you get into the habit of turning things around physically with a walk, you'll start to do the same mentally; this can shift your perception and help you think laterally.

DISCOVERY WALK

This type of walk will help you get to know your neighborhood. Even if you've been living somewhere for years, you might surprise yourself and find a patch with new delights to offer. All you have to do is keep your wits about you, stay present and open, and observe each walkway keenly. You'll need to keep an eye on time as this is only a short stroll, but if you do find something of interest you can always go back for a longer ramble.

- Set yourself a time limit. You may have a destination in mind, but don't be tied to it. Keep in mind that you are going on something of an adventure!
- Adopt a leisurely pace; you don't want to be rushing and miss anything of interest. This is about observing your surroundings and enjoying the sights and sounds that you see every day.
- Take time to appreciate the flowering borders that line the street, noticing how they frame the view with their pretty shapes and colors.
- Admire the sprawling canopy of a particular tree, as well as the intricate pattern of its branches.
- Gaze up into the sky and watch the birds soaring overhead.
- Look down at your feet and notice the contours of the path you are following.

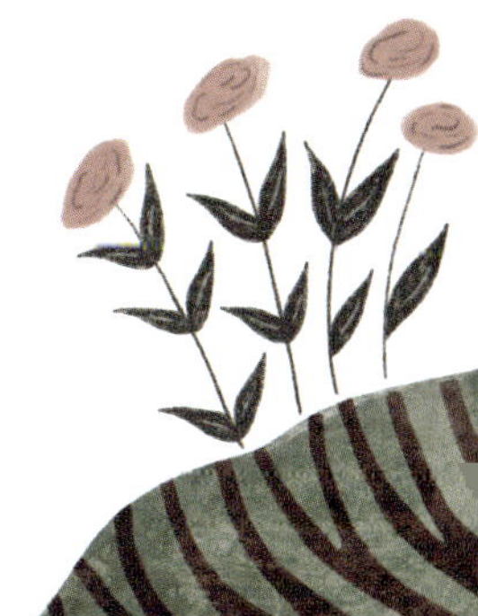

- Survey your surroundings and watch the natural world unfold before your eyes. Even in the most urban environments, nature finds a way to break through. Wildflowers peep between the cracks in paving stones, moss gathers on stone walls, and bushes become homes for small birds, seeking refuge from the noise and bustle of the human world.

- Give yourself the permission and freedom to sightsee and have fun, even if it is for a limited time. In doing so, you'll open the mind and enliven the spirit.

- Look for openings and opportunities to explore—a rusty gate that leads to a tree-lined walkway, an avenue with blooming planters and hanging baskets. It doesn't matter if the route doesn't lead to your destination; you're allowed to be spontaneous and take a diversion.

- If you do find something of interest, make a mental note, so you can return and explore more fully on another day.

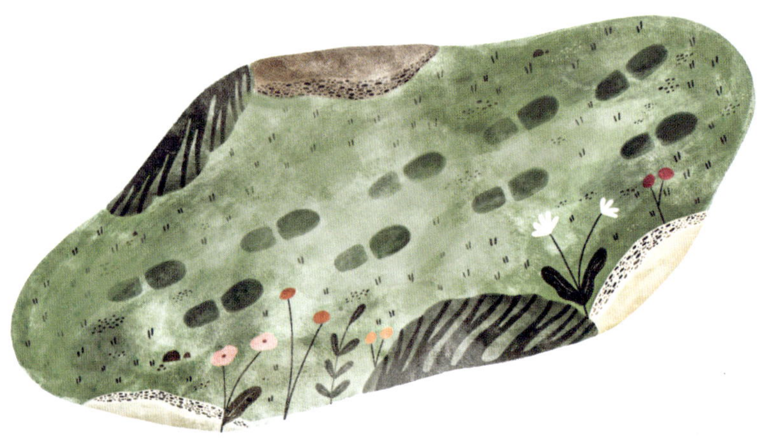

WALK 32

Clear the Path for New Beginnings

A bracing walk on a windy day is an effective way of exercising and ultimately strengthens the body and mind. When you walk into the wind, the resistance you feel forces the muscles to work harder, making it more of a challenge. The effort you put into each step means that a walk around your local park is not dissimilar to a hike across a rugged landscape or walking up a steep hill. Add to this the fact that wind accelerates the evaporation of sweat, which means you'll stay cool and clear-headed for longer, and you have a win-win situation when it comes to fitness and feeling good.

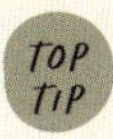

GIVE YOURSELF A PUSH

This is a brisk walk, so you'll need to increase the pace and length of your gait. It's a good idea to build up to this gradually during the walk. The more energized you feel by your surroundings, the more effort you'll put into each step. It helps to imagine that your feet are bouncing forward and that you're cushioned by the air. This will propel you forward and generate even more energy!

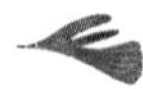

WINDY WALK

If you're looking for a short stroll that will leave you firing on all cylinders, then choose a windy day in spring. The season of new growth and renewal is the perfect time of year to embark on a brisk walk. There's plenty to see and stimulate the senses and the wind will put a spring in your step.

- Find your balance to begin with, so take a minute to stand and let the wind buffet you. Fix your feet on the ground, take a long breath in, and, as you release it, let the weight drop a little into your legs and knees. Tighten your tummy muscles to engage your core and feel centered.

- Stride into the wind as you walk. Your purpose is to work those muscles and let the power of the breeze work against you. Feel the air pushing against your face; feel it whipping around your limbs as you take each step.

- Breathe deeply as you go and imagine the wind stripping you of any stagnant energy. Imagine that each gust is pulling the tension from your body and clearing your head of negative thoughts.

- Engage with your surroundings, so, if you're walking in your local park, make a point of looking for signs of spring. Take note of tiny flower buds that appear in clumps at your feet and around the base of trees. Look at the thickness of the grass, at the new shoots that are bursting through the soil, hungry for a gulp of fresh air. Look up into the trees and see the fresh green leaves that have started to appear, the blossom spilling from the branches in a profusion of white and pink, frothy bundles. Notice how everything seems brighter and more potent with spring's revitalizing energy.

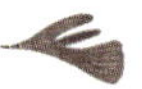

- Imagine that the wind whirling around you carries with it the rejuvenating magic of spring, and that with each step you are heading farther into this force field. Each breath you take imbues you with this vibrant energy. Your head feels clear. Your heart beats with power and vitality. Your body feels strong and energized.
- Put more effort into each step. Stretch your senses even further and embrace the return of the season as you continue on your path.

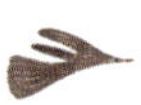

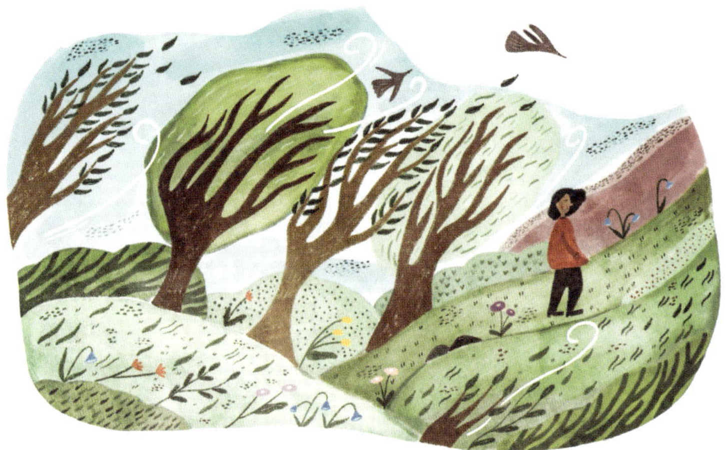

WALK 33

Embrace a Sudden Shower

You might not fancy a short stroll in the rain, but there are lots of reasons why your body and brain will thank you. Rainfall cleanses the air and mind, not to mention the petrichor effect—the pleasant, musky scent that is released as rain water hits dry earth, has a soothing effect on the brain. So, while a rainy walk might not appeal, it's worth making the extra effort to get out there.

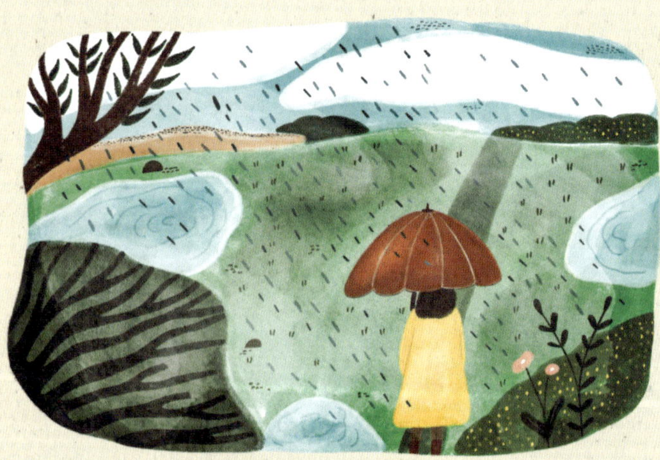

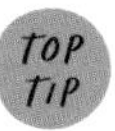

WHAT A WONDERFUL WORLD!

If you're stuck in a rut, embrace the energy of a rainy walk to boost your mood and help you move forward. Treat each puddle as an opportunity to generate movement by stepping wholeheartedly into it. Feel the splash and let the playful excitement of it spur you onward. If you prefer, stride over the puddles with confidence and know that you can do the same with any obstacles you encounter in your path. Let the cool touch of each drop of rain upon your face stimulate the senses and inspire you. Feel the energy bubbling under your skin and smile!

PUDDLE HOPPING

Throw yourself into this type of walk by engaging all your senses. Take a childlike approach and enjoy the refreshing energy of a sudden downpour. Look at your surroundings with fresh eyes, and you will widen your perspective and develop a positive mindset.

- Make sure you prepare before you leave home. You'll need the right clothes, so you can walk with confidence and stay dry. So, invest in some waterproofs, including the appropriate footwear and an umbrella.

- Choose a short, familiar route as rain can make it hard to see when you walk. A short walk to the store or through your local park is ideal. If you have some countryside on your doorstep, then use that, but halve your normal walking route or work out a circular track that brings you back home.

- Walk with purpose. Increase your usual speed and put some energy into each step. Remember how you walked in the rain as a child, splashing in puddles or jumping over them, and recreate that sense of wonder. Embrace the joy of the splash, and notice how you feel when your feet enter the water. Breathe quickly and deeply, taking in deep lungfuls of air and purging them from your body with a replenishing sigh. This will keep your energy level high and motivate you to continue.

- Engage your other senses. Notice how the rain washes over everything, giving the color palette depth and brightness. See how the grass shines a deep emerald green and the sidewalks glisten like steely rivers at your feet. Pay attention to the flowers and see how they bend under the weight of each raindrop, the hues of the petals gleaming like jewels. Inhale the fresh aroma of the rainfall and follow the scent. Let it lift your spirits and lead you onward.

- Be confident with each step you take. Don't shy away from the rain; open yourself up to it instead. Listen to the rain's gentle patter and let it wash over you. Imagine that the raindrops are cleansing you from head to toe, clearing the path for new and exciting opportunities.

- Once you reach your destination, dry yourself off and reflect upon your walk. Did you enjoy it more than you thought and how do you feel now?

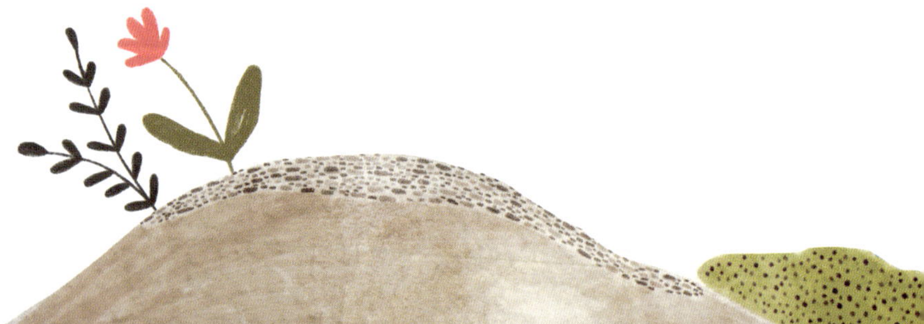

WALK 34

Get Out in the Garden

If you have some outdoor space, then make the most of it by taking a short daily walk. You might spend time sitting in your garden with friends and family, but a walk is an entirely different experience. It gives you a unique viewpoint of a space that you know well.

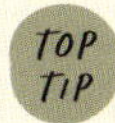

FIND YOUR SPACE

If you don't have your own garden, why not borrow someone else's outdoor space. Perhaps you have an elderly neighbor or relative that needs help looking after theirs. If so, volunteer your services, then you'll have regular access to green space. If you prefer, you can visit open gardens near you. The space you find doesn't have to be massive; a small area is all you need for an inspirational stroll to boost creativity.

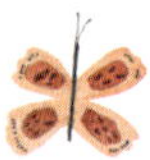

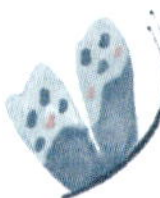

SURVEILLANCE STROLL

You may think you know your garden, but there are plenty of nooks and crannies that can be easily missed. Tiny spaces are busy hubs for small invertebrates, while flower bushes provide a home to a range of winged wonders.

Use this walk to survey your environment thoroughly. Take in the details and look at each section from a different perspective. In doing so, you'll discover the hidden gems at your fingertips, while stretching your legs and getting regular exercise. You'll also boost your innate creativity, and you may even come up with new ideas to help your garden work for you and the creatures that live there.

STEP 1 *Start at one end of the garden and work out a circular path* that allows you to walk close to borders and fences or hedges. If the space isn't particularly big, you can do this a few times, taking your time on the first appraisal and then picking up speed at each turn.

STEP 2 *Imagine you're a visitor to the garden for the first time*. What are your initial impressions? How does the sight of the garden make you feel? What do you love about it? What could you change?

STEP 3 *Pay close attention* to the bushes and shrubs that line the garden and look along hedges and fences to see what catches your eye.

STEP 4 *Seek out movement* and see how many creatures you can spot. You might not see anything at first, which is why you'll need to walk around the space a few times. Each time you'll notice something different.

STEP 5 *Stop by a flowering bush and take in its beauty.* Notice movement and sound, and check for bees or other pollinators.

STEP 6 *Take a long, deep breath in.* What can you smell?

STEP 7 *Look for spaces that need to be filled,* and think about the types of flowers and shrubs you could plant that might attract more pollinators.

STEP 8 *Continue on your journey,* paying attention to what is at your feet and also what is overhead.

STEP 9 *Look down and check for animal tracks.* Are there spaces for animals and insects to congregate? A compost pile? A bug hotel? Even a stack of wood could create a safe haven for any number of small creatures.

STEP 10 *Look up and turn around.* What can you see? How does the garden look from higher up. Do you have bird or bee boxes or perhaps a bird table?

STEP 11 *Take in every little detail as you walk,* then repeat the process at least two or three more times.

STEP 12 *Let your imagination take over* and let ideas rise to the surface. Looking at this space in a new way will stimulate your innate creativity, so you might feel the urge to sketch, write, or simply list some ideas when you're done.

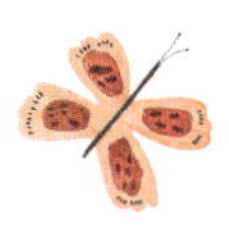

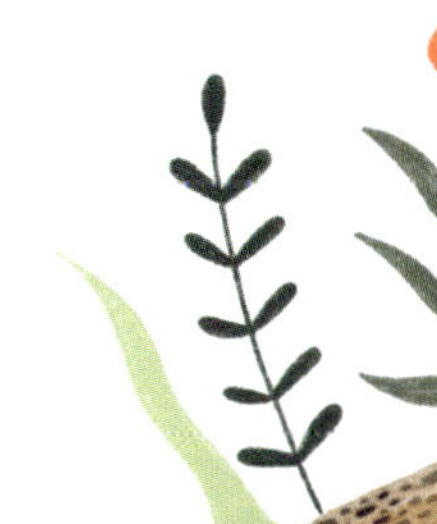

WALK 35

Give Yourself a Lunchtime Lift

Your lunch break is an excellent opportunity for a breather. A short, relaxing walk at this time will break up the day and banish stress. Evidence suggests regular walking improves cardiovascular health, and according to research, women who take a thirty-minute walk every day can reduce their risk of a stroke by twenty percent (a figure which increases to forty percent if the pace is increased). Combine this with the mental health benefits of an improved mood and self-esteem, and the fact that walking adds structure to a busy workday, and there's no excuse not to enjoy a lunchtime stroll.

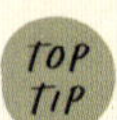

COMMUNE WITH A TREE

If your walk allows, find a big tree like an oak and take five minutes to sit beneath its boughs. Press the base of your spine into the ground, then gently lean back and let the trunk support you. Place your hands in your lap and drink in your surroundings. Imagine that you are infused by the stoic strength of this tree. Feel the energy travel along your spine, each time you inhale. Use this time to relax in any way you want. For example, you might want to close your eyes, daydream, or read a book before returning to work.

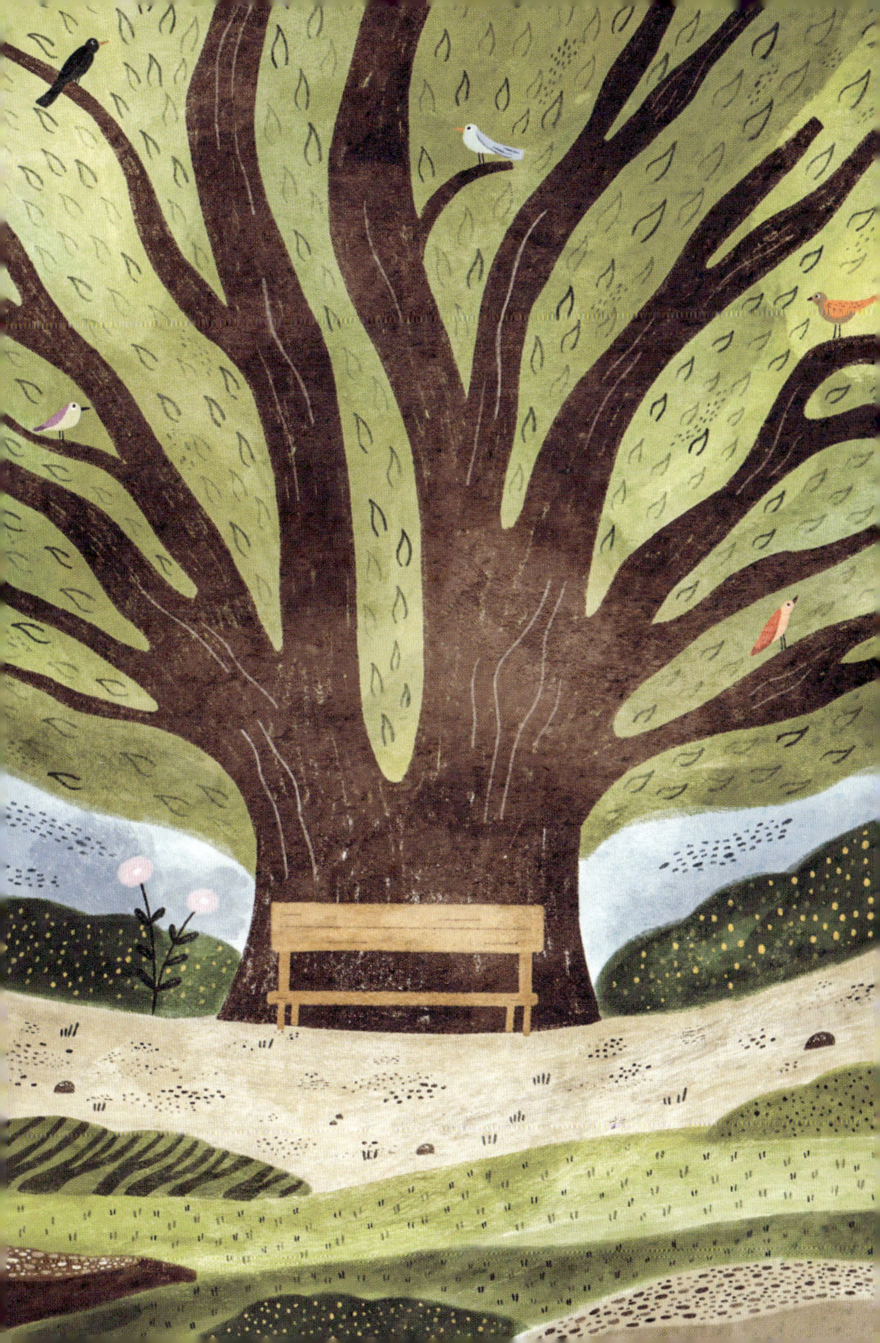

A LUNCHTIME RESET

Most of us rush through our lunch break, trying to fit in hundreds of things before returning to work where we are faced with even more stress. Instead, use the time for a steady walk that allows you breathing space and the opportunity to check in with yourself and where you are, in the present moment.

STEP 1 *If possible, find some green space* that you can appreciate, so find a garden, park, or cemetery that you can wander through. This walk is about slowing down and allowing your body and mind to breathe, so take your time.

STEP 2 *Position each foot carefully* on the ground and feel the earth anchoring every step you take.

STEP 3 *Breathe deeply and let your body relax.* Release tension from your shoulders by rolling them back and down and let your arms swing naturally by your sides. Take fluid steps from the hip, feeling the weight gradually move into your knees and calves.

STEP 4 *Pause and take in your surroundings.* What can you see? What catches your eye? Perhaps the movement of a bird foraging in the grass or the leaves on the trees dancing in the breeze. Let this moment capture your attention fully and focus only on what you can see around you.

STEP 5 *If any thoughts about work stress arise, don't hold on to them.* Instead, return your attention to the natural beauty of the environment, and let this fill your mind instead.

STEP 6 *Use this moment to check in with yourself.* How do you feel right now, physically and emotionally?

STEP 7 *Acknowledge any feelings or sensations, but don't hold on to them.* Instead, let them go by taking a long, cleansing breath, up through the soles of your feet, along your legs, and into your torso and chest, and then releasing it slowly through pursed lips.

STEP 8 *Continue on your way,* letting the environment soothe you as you go.

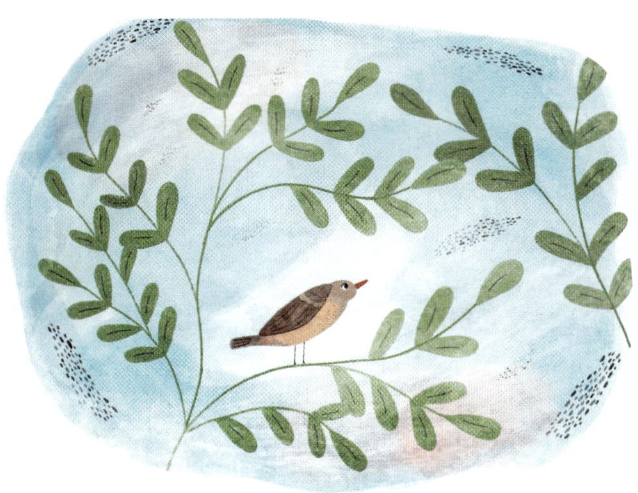

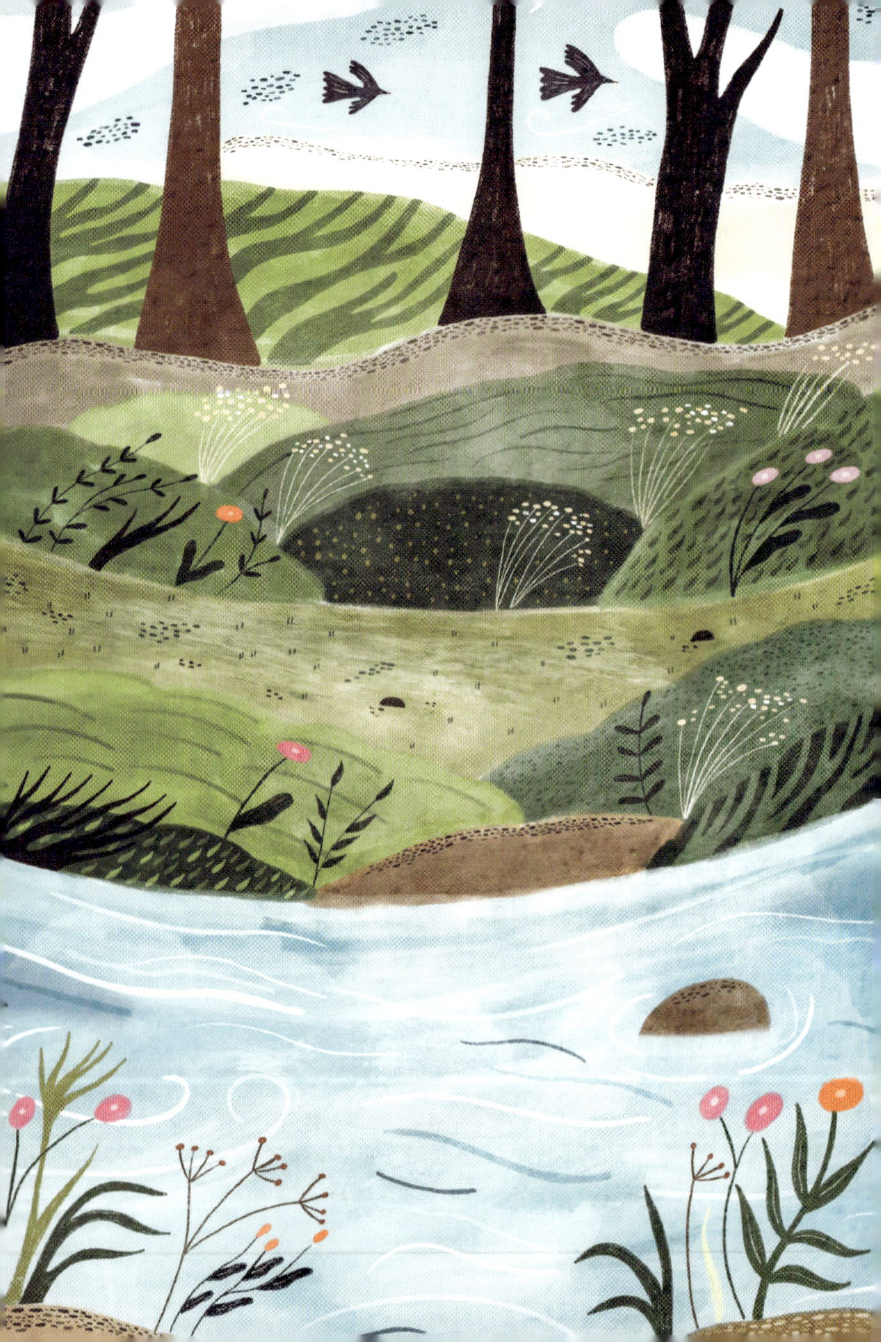

CHAPTER FIVE

Walking BY Waterways

The tranquility of a waterway stroll cannot be matched. The soothing setting, combined with a plethora of sights, sounds, and smells, makes a waterside setting the perfect backdrop for any type of walk. Whether you're in search of peace, or looking to clear away the cobwebs and feel invigorated, you'll find what you need here.

WALK 36

Go with the Flow

Research suggests that spending time near bodies of water, known as "blue spaces," has a calming effect on mental health. The movement of the water, together with the soothing sounds of the flow, lulls the mind, alleviates stress, and helps us feel more positive.

Rivers, streams, and other natural bodies of water are synonymous with fun, conjuring up memories of happy times spent outside. Make the most of this uplifting energy with a relaxing riverside stroll to release anxiety.

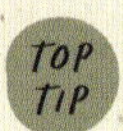

WATER UNDER THE BRIDGE

If you're lucky enough to come across a bridge during your river stroll, make the most of it. Use this space to release anything that is holding you back into the flow of water beneath you, and then set intentions for the future. You'll need something light enough to float away, like a feather or some flower petals. Hold your offering in both hands and close your eyes for a moment. Think about the future and what you'd like to create. Sum this up in a simple sentence that captures the essence of your wish. For example, you might be hoping to move house and start again in a new location, so you might say, "I manifest new opportunities to broaden my horizons and start afresh." Drop your offering over the edge of the bridge and watch as it is carried forward by the flowing water.

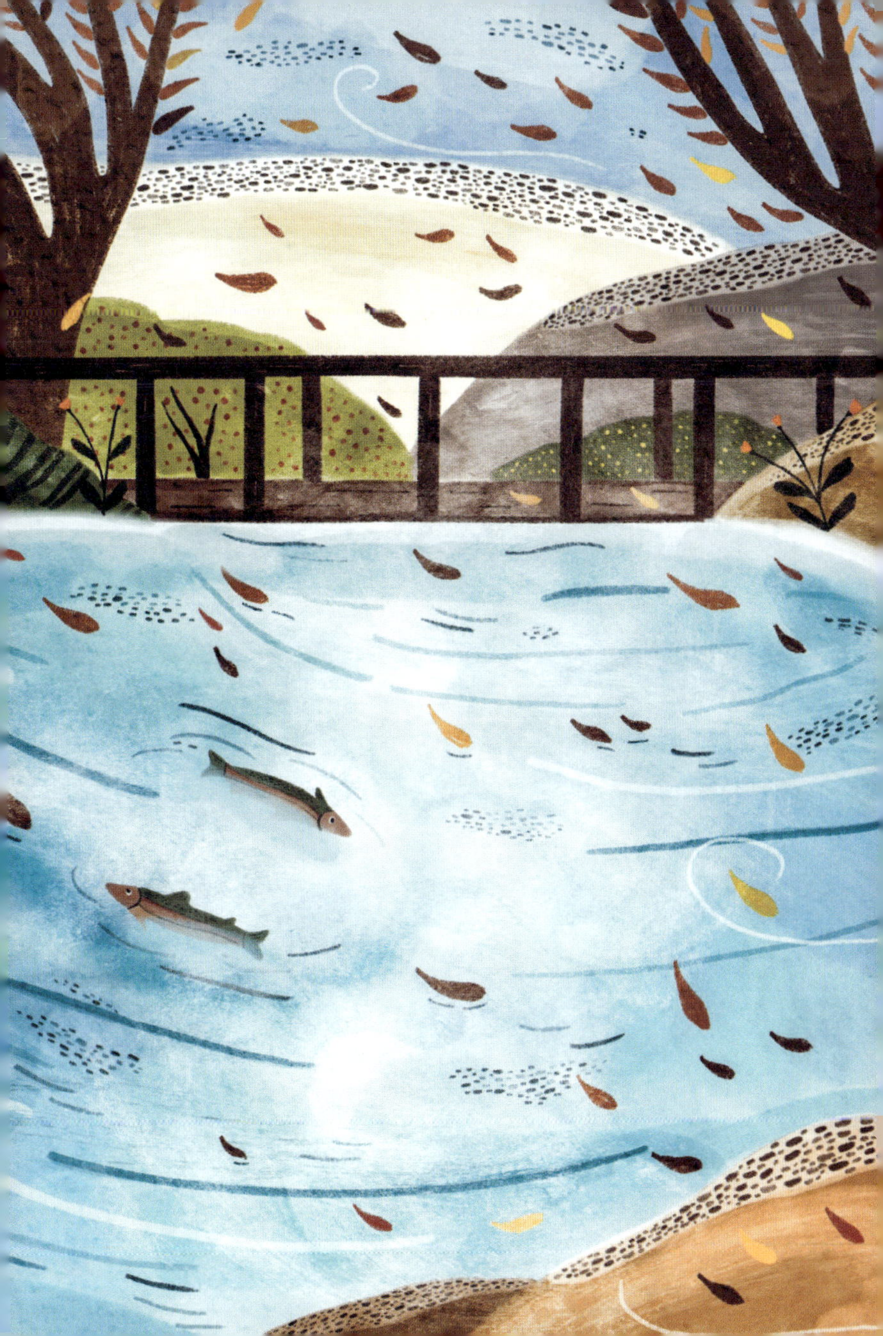

LETTING GO AS YOU WALK

Any body of water works for this exercise, which combines the natural flow of water with the gentle motion of a walk. You can do this at any point in the year, but the chill of a winter setting will encourage you to go within, reflect, and release what you no longer need. Spring is also an opportune time to recharge and release the past. The joyful sight of flower buds coming into bloom promotes positive energy, which can help when letting go of negative thought patterns.

You will need a stretch of water that is fairly long, and one where you can walk close to the riverbank, but at a safe distance. The most important thing is to enjoy this stroll and treat it as an act of self-care. This is not about breaking into a sweat or covering a lot of ground, but about taking your time, reflecting, and reveling in nature's beauty.

STEP 1 *Walk at a steady pace*, and relax your shoulders and arms. Let them fall naturally by your sides. Give your body the freedom to move as it wishes.

STEP 2 *Engage your senses as you stroll.* Listen to the rhythmic pulse of your heartbeat and the way your feet sound as they take each step. Listen to the breeze through the shrubs and trees, and the gentle music it makes. Most importantly, listen out for the sound of the water as it trickles onward. Notice any changes in the sound that the river makes, from the whooshing as it picks up pace to the babbling noise as it rushes over rocks and stones. Listen for the sounds of nature—for example, a group of geese dipping their beaks beneath the surface of the water, or a swan ruffling its feathers as it alights on the riverbank. Watch the steady flow of the water, and let it mesmerize you.

STEP 3 *As you walk, keep your eyes peeled for the gifts of nature*, such as a beautiful feather or stone, or a pretty flower head lying at your feet. Find an object that you are drawn to and pick it up. Take a moment to stand by the river and take in its beauty.

STEP 4 *Hold the object in your hands,* and think about all the things that you would like to release from your life. For example, you might carry guilt or fear, or have a habit that you'd like to let go of.

STEP 5 *Take a deep breath* in and, as you exhale, imagine pouring all these negative emotions into the object you found.

STEP 6 *Take another deep, cleansing breath,* and as you exhale let the object fall into the river. Release it from your grasp and say either out loud or in your head, "I release with love what I no longer need. I let the river cleanse my body, mind, and soul."

STEP 7 *Watch the flow of the water,* and know that life always moves on and that you too can carry on moving forward.

STEP 8 *Continue enjoying your riverside stroll* and absorbing the peaceful atmosphere of this place.

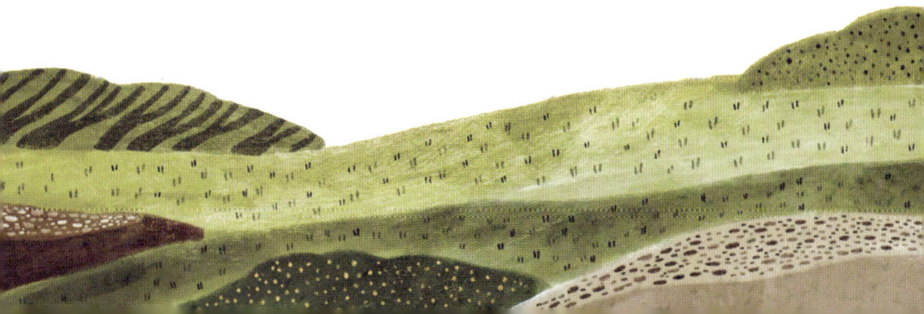

WALK 37

Cleanse and Recharge

Being in the presence of a waterfall is a truly inspiring experience; the power of the cascade stirs the soul. The sound of a waterfall also has a "white noise" effect, and together these provide a natural phenomenon that inspires and soothes in equal measure.

Waterfalls are an abundant source of negative ions, also known as "air vitamins." These invisible molecules are odorless and are thought to have a positive effect on health, reducing stress levels, boosting mood and energy, and improving the metabolism.

Some waterfalls are human-made, while others are shaped by Mother Nature and are the result of natural erosion, as river water surges over rock to find its own tumbling path. It doesn't matter which kind you happen to find on a ramble, you'll reap the benefits, especially if you're looking for a natural way to recharge.

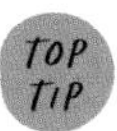

LET THE FALLS INSPIRE YOU

Waterfalls have been a source of inspiration and creativity for thousands of years. Poets, writers, and artists have been continually captivated by their beauty. Ancient civilizations revered them, believing they could cleanse the soul of bad luck and promote the flow of wealth. Consider this while taking a waterfall walk. Give your imagination free rein and come up with an artistic interpretation of the waterfall, either by scribbling a poem or sketching it.

EMBRACE THE CASCADE

Whether the waterfall is big or small, it is imbued with magical energy. Simply taking in the sight is enough to calm the mind, but to really appreciate the waterfall effect, you'll need to get up close and personal and feel the spray of water.

- Do your research. Get to know the walks that might feature waterfalls, so you're likely to encounter one. It's a joy to stumble upon this phenomenon spontaneously, but if you're going out with the intention of connecting with this natural beauty, then this will increase your chances of success.

- Make sure you're wearing appropriate clothing like waterproof clothes and boots. When choosing footwear, go with something that has a good grip as you might find that rocks and paths are slippery.

- The prelude to reaching the waterfall is the ideal time to exercise your senses, so make sure you take in everything you can see, hear, smell, and touch.

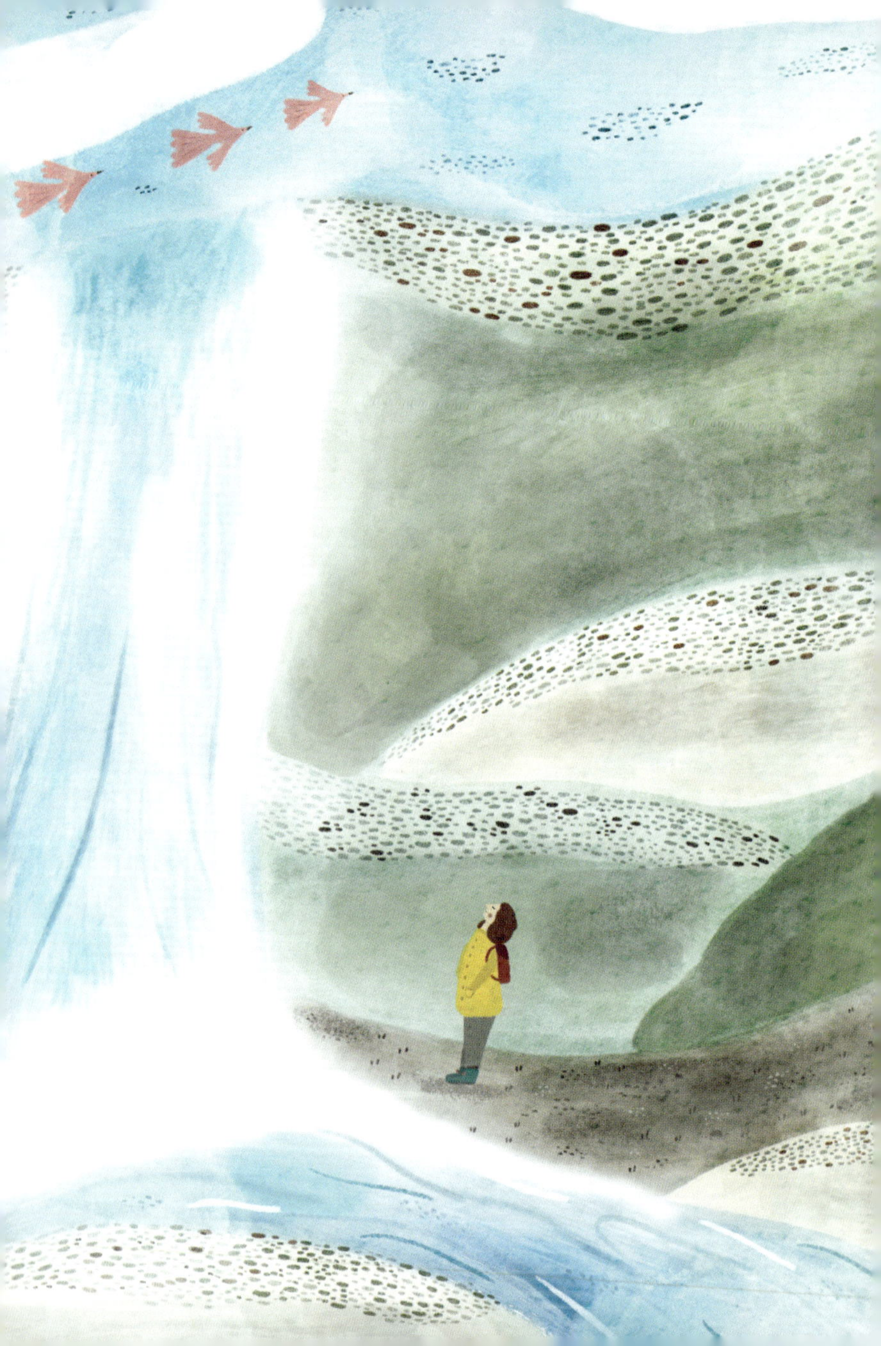

- Once in the presence of the waterfall, take a minute to appreciate its beauty. Stand and breathe deeply. Imagine you're watching a performance and absorb every detail, from the silvery, flowing water to the whooshing sound it makes as it surges over the edge.

- If you can do so safely, get close to the waterfall. Stand within arm's reach of the spray and stretch out your fingers. Feel the delicate touch of the droplets as they dance on your skin. Close your eyes and really focus on this feeling. If you feel brave enough, and it's possible, you might be able to stand beneath the arch of the water, but if not, stand where you are and imagine that you are beneath the cascading water.

- Imagine the sensation as the water hits the top of your head and sprays outward, showering you in refreshing rivulets. Feel the purity of the spray surging over you. Feel it cleansing every part of your body. Take a long, deep breath in, and as you exhale, imagine the water rushing through you like a river of vibrant white energy. Take this revitalizing feeling with you, as you continue on your route.

Find the Source

Humans have been drawn to water throughout history. For early tribes, it was essential for survival, and settlements were often built close to rivers and lakes for this reason. Ancient peoples performed elaborate rituals involving water. They made sacrifices to the gods and petitioned them for rain, but, most importantly, they believed in its sacred nature, believing it was synonymous with purity. They recognized the power of standing by free-flowing water and taking in its beauty.

Today, we know that the presence of water stimulates the parasympathetic nervous system, helping us to relax, but like those who came before us, we can also appreciate its magnificence—the awe-inspiring sight of a surging river, the peaceful serenity of a lake on a summer's day, or the playful trickle of a mountain stream.

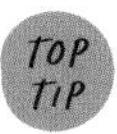

CHANNEL YOUR POSITIVITY

With the positive mindset you gain from this walk, why not take things a step further. During your next walk think of all the things that you are grateful for in your life, so, for every gift of nature, find something in your own life to be thankful for. Give thanks silently in your head or out loud if you want to. Embrace the positivity and the joy of gratitude. The magical combination of acknowledging Mother Nature's gifts, walking at a brisk pace, and being near water will help you feel energized and should boost your mood at the same time!

GRATITUDE WALK

Use the canvas of a walk along your favorite river or lake to build a gratitude list which will put you in a positive mindset. If you open your heart and mind as you walk, and look at your surroundings with fresh eyes, you will notice a myriad of natural blessings all around you.

This walk is all about enjoying yourself, so set a brisk, proactive pace to lift the heart rate and boost your mood. It doesn't matter what time of year you choose for this walk. Each season has something to offer, and it can be uplifting to do this when the weather isn't at its best because it proves that even on the darkest days we can find something to be thankful for.

STEP 1 *As you begin walking, remember to keep your eyes peeled* and let nature take its course. You will find that all sorts of things capture your attention, from the flurry of movement in a clump of grass to a swan gliding along the surface of the water.

STEP 2 *Take note of each thing you spot, and find something positive to say about it;* for example, you might admire the duck's graceful movement or the way the wind makes the reeds dance. You might notice the sharp smell of the hedgerow, the fresh aromatic fragrance of herbs, or the earthy smell of the mud at your feet. You might hear a blackbird singing in the distance or be startled by the squawking of a gaggle of geese. Every sight, sound, smell, and feeling offers something to value.

STEP 3 *Each time you notice and appreciate something, take a minute to say thank you* in your head. Acknowledge the wonders of nature and be grateful for these gifts.

STEP 4 *When you reach the end of your walk, repeat this affirmation* with feeling. Say, "I am thankful for the joy of this walk, for the blessings of nature, and for everything I have seen and experienced."

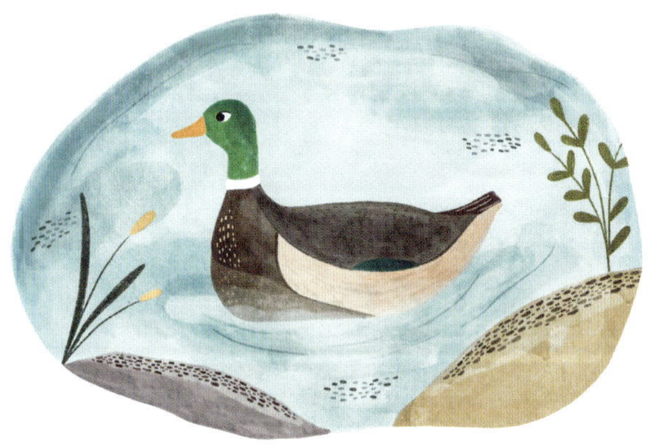

WALK 39

Find Your Path

Water always finds its way. The flow of a river is not easily tamed, for while it may hit obstacles like rocks and boulders, it always finds a path over or around them. There's a flexibility about the way it surges onward, taking a new direction to reach its desired destination. Take inspiration from this and let nature help you find your way.

DIP YOUR HANDS IN THE WATER

If you can get near the edge of the stream safely, bend down and dip your hands into the glistening water. Feel the coolness filtering between your fingers; feel it gently touching your skin as the stream trickles onward. Notice how the water calms and supports you. Imagine the refreshing liquid washing your hands, so they tingle with invigorating energy. Visualize the water flowing gradually up each arm, moving through your entire body until you are cleansed from head to toe. Sit with this rejuvenating energy for a moment and let it wash over you.

BLUE SPACE THINKING

Walking by water is a great leveler. It helps you find perspective and provides the clear, open space needed to see a way forward. It's the perfect time to reflect on your life and give yourself some breathing space.

When we are immersed in the beauty of nature, we often come up with the best solutions to problems. The natural surroundings, fresh air, and injection of blue space work together to induce creative flow.

Before you begin this walk, set the intention that you are going to clear your mind and aim to come up with the inspiration you need to move forward. While it's tempting to focus solely on the issue that you need help with, try not to dwell on it. Instead, you're going to use this restorative time to empty your mind and think creatively.

You'll need to look out for stretches of countryside with natural sources of water, so hillside streams with tiny rivulets of water that meander downward are ideal.

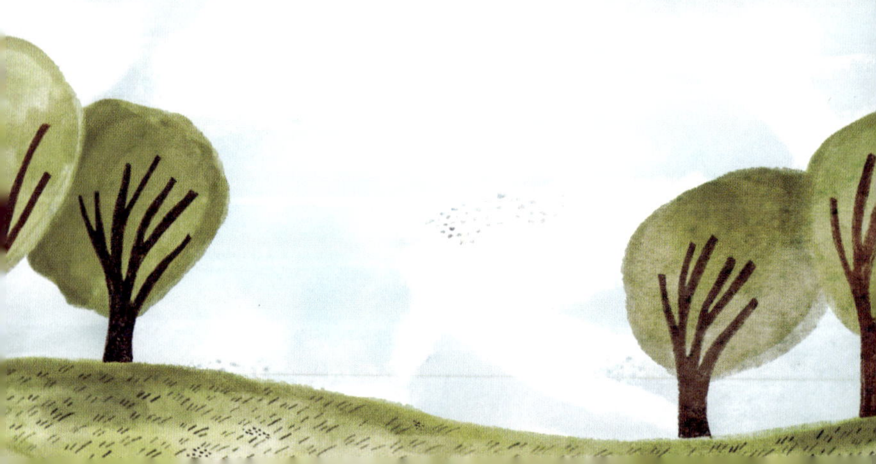

STEP 1 *When you find a stream,* even if it's just a tiny trickle, follow its path with your eyes. If you can walk beside it safely, then do so.

STEP 2 *Notice how the stream carves a path through the earth,* falling easily over or around rocks and stony areas. Think about the ways in which you too have been like this stream and found a new path in life. Consider your journey so far and how you've evolved.

STEP 3 *Bring to mind past challenges that you have overcome.* When you were faced with an obstacle, did you take a new path and work your way around it? If so, how did this work out for you?

STEP 4 *Bring your attention back to the stream and take a minute to appreciate its journey.* Does the stream split into two separate directions or change direction completely? Notice that this doesn't halt its passage. If anything, this makes the flow stronger.

STEP 5 *Is there a way that you can take another path* or change direction with your current issue?

STEP 6 *Drink in the tranquil progress of the water as it works its way downhill.* Know that whatever direction you choose to take, you are still moving forward. Your current challenge will soon be a moment in your past. Like the stream that rolls onward, life continues to flow and you will find a way through this situation.

WALK 40

Winter Wanderings

There's a shift in brightness, with the arrival of winter. While some environments appear stark and gray, bodies of water like lakes and rivers take on a dazzling hue. Skies thicken with snow, their beauty reflected upon the surface of the water. The wide-open spaces expand even more to give a clear view of any wildlife. Areas of natural beauty tend to be quieter at this time of year too, so you'll have the opportunity to see more.

This is the season of drama, of theatrical vistas and cool, crisp air. If you're looking to clear your mind of clutter, take a river walk during the colder months and make the most of the season's gifts.

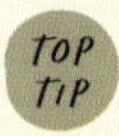

CREATIVITY IN THE COLD

This type of dramatic vista is inspiring and can stimulate your creative brain. Why not put pen to paper and write a poem, or make a few notes on your phone? Start by taking in what you can see and compare it to earlier in the year. Think about the things that stand out, the highlights of your walk, and write a few words to describe them. Take some photos along the way, so you can refer back to them and really explore your creative side when you get home in the warmth of your home.

WINTER RIVER RAMBLE

Clear the cobwebs with a brisk winter walk. Increase your usual strolling speed and take in your surroundings as you go. Make sure you are wrapped up warm for this walk. The wind that blows over water picks up more moisture, giving it an icy feel, so wear plenty of layers and the right footwear. You'll need strong, supportive boots with a good grip, as the ground may be slippery underfoot.

- Before you begin, take a moment to adjust your vision. Close your eyes and feel the cool air on your skin. Take a long, deep breath in and, as you exhale, slowly open your eyes. Let them become accustomed to the light, which is often brighter at this time of year.
- Look ahead and focus on something in the distance, then let your awareness expand to take in the river by your side.
- As you walk, drink in the view. Notice the frost-dappled trees and the skeletal branches that border the water's edge. Take in the colors, the silvery shrubs, and ethereal bushes that line the path and the looming shapes of the trees in the distance. It's a very different landscape from those earlier spring and summer rambles.
- Breathe deeply and let the cold air fill your lungs. Imagine that with each breath, you are infusing your brain with this cooling energy. Draw in this energy and let it permeate your being.
- Let the power of the landscape banish any self-doubt and silence negative thoughts.
- Repeat this affirmation in your head as you walk, "Every step I take, I feel brighter and lighter."

WALK 41

Go Forth and Forage

Foraging walks are a popular way to get to know an area, and learn about edible plants, fungi, and other natural resources. While woodland settings are the usual choice for this type of ramble, a waterway walk also has much to offer. You can take your time, appreciate the landscape as you go, and benefit from the steady serenity of the water.

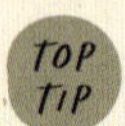

MAKE A FORAGED MEMENTO

Keep the non-edible items you've collected and have a go at creating a collage or decoration with them when you get home. This can be anything from a simple table display in a decorative bowl to something more elaborate, if you're feeling artistic. If you prefer, you can use them to stimulate your creativity, by sketching them or letting your imagination take over and writing something inspired by your finds. Whatever you come up with, it's a memento of your walk.

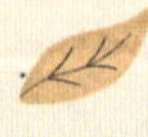
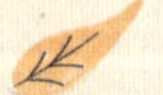
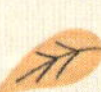
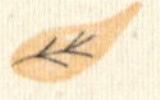
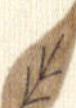

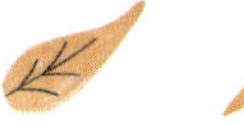

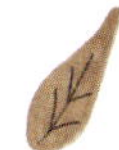

SCAVENGER WALK

Anything goes when you're scavenging—it's about finding those gifts of nature that catch your eye. This type of walk is immersive and offers you the opportunity to really connect with the environment, which enriches your experience.

- Enjoy the walk as you would normally, but keep your eye out for any forage-friendly items. When you find something that you think looks interesting, be sure to check it out either by using a handy pocket guide or on your phone. The general rule is don't pick anything that you can't identify, and always wash plants before you eat them.

- If you're scavenging for interesting non-edible finds, be sure to look beneath the surface, so under plants and bushes, down at the side of the riverbank, or along the towpath.

- Set yourself a challenge to find at least three different items that you can take back with you after your walk. This will help to fire up your observation skills.

You can scavenge for anything, depending on where you are. Here's a list of things to look for on your walk, based on location.

CANALS
Look out for edibles like blackberries, elderberries, damsons, watermint, chickweed, rosehips, sloe berries, crab apples, and nettles. You may also find dandelions or other edible wildflowers.

RIVERS AND LAKES
Look out for watercress and coltsfoot, and also chicken of the woods, a mushroom that is often found growing beneath willow trees on riverbanks.

WALK 42

Survey Your Surroundings

A reservoir walk is the ideal environment to hone your observation skills. This type of walk is structured, and if it's somewhere you go on a regular basis, you'll get to know what to expect at various locations along the way. With this in mind, you'll be able to note any changes and also pay attention to the different types of wildlife.

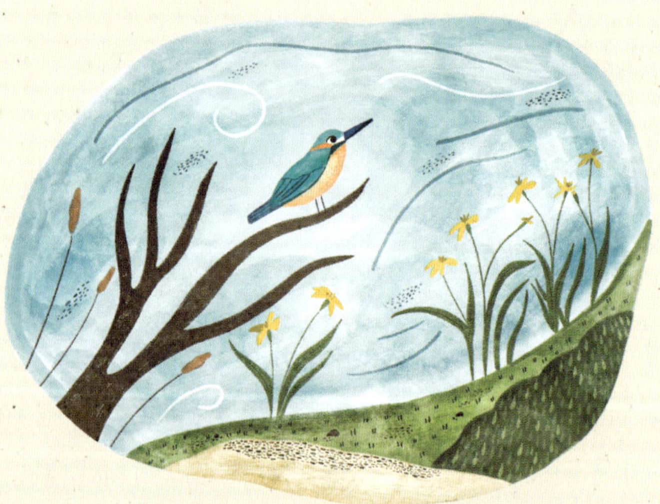

FIND YOUR FOCUS

Put your keen observation skills to the test and record everything you see as you walk. To help with this, keep a notebook with you or make notes on your phone. A quick description of what you see, including where you saw it, will help you make an identification when you return home.

Keeping a log of what you see, and when, will also inform future walks. For example, if you fancy catching sight of a particular bird and you know it tends to surface during the summer months, you'll have more chance of seeing it then. If you have a particular area of interest—for example, birds or insects—it's a good idea to take a pocket-sized guide with you, so you can refer to it when you need it. What to look out for:

- A natural stronghold for many birds, including ducks, geese, swans, grebes, cormorants, coots, and a variety of gulls, reservoirs are a rich opportunity for birdwatchers. Songbirds like thrushes and redpolls can often be seen in scrub and grassland near large bodies of water.

- Reservoirs are also the place to go if you want to observe flora and fauna through the seasons, as you'll be able to see distinct shifts in the landscape and record these changes.

- Mammals are in abundance in this type of environment, so look out for otters, bats, squirrels, and voles, along with amphibians like toads, newts, and frogs.

- The freshwater environment is ideal for a variety of fish to thrive. Even if you're not a keen angler, spotting the fish weaving beneath the surface as you take a steady stroll is incredibly rewarding. Look out for carp, trout, bream, and roach. Pike are also prevalent in many reservoirs, on the hunt for smaller fish to satisfy their large appetites!

WALK 43

Water Scrying

Water has been used for thousands of years as a tool to divine the future. The ancient Greeks were particular proponents, and would often use pools of water for this purpose. This practice, known as scrying, involved gazing into the surface of the water to induce a trance-like state. The scryer would then wait for patterns and symbols to emerge on the surface. The famous astrologer and physician Nostradamus was a huge advocate. He kept a scrying bowl on hand for his predictions.

Today, we gaze into water to still the mind and promote peaceful feelings. According to science, the sight and sound of flowing water triggers the release of neurochemicals in the brain, which lower stress hormones like cortisol, so while you might not wish to divine the future, you'll still gain inspiration, strength, and clarity from this practice.

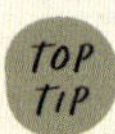

SURFACES FOR REFLECTION

You can use the natural backdrop of any walk as a focal point to soothe your mind. Water is easy to use because it is reflective, and waterways offer an array of features that can stimulate or still the mind. But look for other natural sources too. A tree stump, with its many-ringed surface, provides an intriguing center for your thoughts, while you breathe deeply to calm your soul.

MIRROR, MIRROR

If you're walking by a stream, river, or pond, stop and take a moment to reflect. Gaze at the surface, and let the calming properties of the water clear your mind and promote inspiration for the future.

STEP 1 *Let your gaze fall upon the water,* and take in the vista as a whole. Notice the gentle movement of the surface: the serene flow that goes ever onward.

STEP 2 *You might catch sight of a water bird*—a wader or a duck floating on the surface. Watch its graceful journey and focus on the steady movement, letting it relax your body and mind.

STEP 3 *When you are ready, take a step closer to the water, so you can see the surface* in front of you more clearly. The water might be murky and full of shadows, or glittering from the sun's light. Focus on what you can see, and if your mind begins to drift, bring it back to the surface of the water.

STEP 4 *You might notice shapes swirling as you gaze deeper,* or even catch sight of a silvery scaled fish. You might see the reflection of the trees or even an impression of your own face. Let the shapes and patterns form and fade.

STEP 5 *Enjoy this space and simply be in the moment,* appreciating what is before you. Take a long, deep breath in, exhale slowly, and relax.

WALK 44

Down the Towpath

The word "canal" comes from the old French term *chanel* meaning "channel." These human-made waterways have played a key role throughout history, especially during the Industrial Revolution when they helped transport goods and exports, which furthered the growth of a number towns and shaped the landscape in new ways. The earliest known examples of canals date back to 2400 BCE, and they were used for irrigation in Mesopotamia.

Today canals are a riot of color and movement. Lined with prettily decorated barges and boats, the dusty towpaths that border the water's edge are littered with sweet-smelling herbs and flowers, an array of wildlife, and more than a few dog walkers, making them the perfect backdrop for ramblers who like to explore.

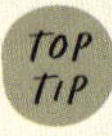

THE BEAUTY OF BARGES

The vibrant and characterful barges on a canal offer plenty of variety during a towpath walk. Each one is unique, from their painted doors and windows to their brightly daubed names. Check out each one and admire its quirky charm. Enjoy this display as if you were perusing the artwork in a famous gallery. It adds a magical element to your walk and will always be different, as the canalside is a shifting, changing landscape.

MINDFUL, MAGICAL, MEDITATIVE MEANDER

Towpaths are a festival for the senses. There's so much to see and experience, and there's a sense of wonder too, a feeling of being one step away from the real world, as you stroll by the water's edge. This landscape is ideal if you want to disconnect from daily stresses and submerge yourself in the magic of nature.

STEP 1 *Being open and present will help you fully appreciate this type of walk.* As you step along the towpath, imagine you've entered another world, slipped between the layers of time and space, and stepped away from the hustle and bustle of life. Switch off your phone, turn off your headphones, and let nature's orchestra take you on a journey.

STEP 2 *With your eyes and ears, pinpoint the steady lap of the water*, the serene ripples that appear on the surface as the canal moves slowly by your side. This is your walking partner and the only distraction you need as

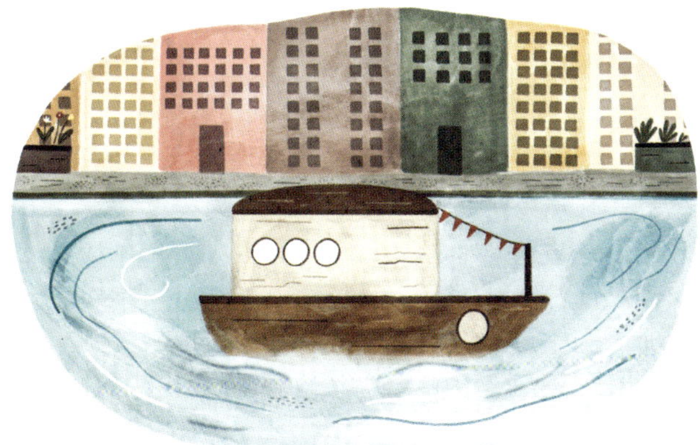

you stride forward. Gradually let other sounds filter through—the tweeting of birds in the distance, the muffled sound of a road on the horizon—background noise that seems far removed from your current location.

STEP 3 *Tap into your inner child as you view your surroundings.* Take in the tall reedy grasses that line the side of the canal and watch them wave in the breeze. Let your fingers caress the tips of the grassy verge and feel the feathery softness against your skin. Breathe deeply and smell the rich aroma of umbellifers and nettles. Elderflower bushes add delicate clusters of powdery whiteness to this scene, while the wild irises and dog roses bunch together, their bright pinks and golds decorating the path. Jewel-like dragonflies dance between leafy fronds near the surface of the water.

STEP 4 *Pick out the curiosities.* Look for the discarded things that have been left behind: pieces of wood and metal from boats that were once moored here; winding paths that lead away from the canal and open up to tree-lined vistas; overhanging bushes that have stood the test of time and droop over the water's edge. They all have a place and a story to tell. Let you imagination piece together their narrative as you stroll.

STEP 5 *Engage with the environment.* You are no longer an onlooker; you are a part of this magical place, so get involved. Sniff the flowers and touch their delicate petals. Smile and wave to the boaters and greet four-legged friends who might wander by and want to say hello. Talk to the bees as they search for pollen and gaze hopefully into the water with a wish in your mind.

WALK 45

Slow Your Flow

There's scientific evidence that the presence of water calms body and mind. The continuous flow and softly lapping sounds act as "white noise," and induces a trance-like state for some people. The fluidity of movement provides an anchor for meditation, encouraging an awareness of the flow of breath in the body and the natural rhythm of the heart. Symbolically, water is associated with "letting go." The graceful flow triggers a primal need to slow down, as we become one with our surroundings.

FIND YOUR BREATH

You don't always have to be on the move. If you find it hard to focus on your breathing as you walk, take a minute to pause. Find a tree by the side of the river or lake; a beautiful overhanging willow with a waterfall of leaves is the perfect spot for a little breathwork. Sit beneath its boughs and press your bottom into the ground. Let your back rest against the trunk of the tree, and feel that gentle support. Let your gaze settle on the flow of the water and begin to breathe deeply, following the journey of each breath and visualizing it in your mind.

WATERWAY MEDITATION WALK

Engage with the environment and use it as a prompt for some breathwork. Take the opportunity as you walk to perform a calming meditation, which focuses on the journey of your breath and the natural flow of the water.

- Focus on your steps, on the natural rhythm of your gait. If you're a fast walker, slow things down a little. Bring your attention to each foot as it connects with the path. Let it sink into the earth, heel to toe.

- Roll your shoulders back and let your arms fall naturally at your sides. Expand your chest and tilt your chin slightly upward by elongating your spine. Feel the gentle stretch. It helps here to imagine a thread traveling up through your back and neck and out of the top of your head, lightly tugging you upward.

- Turn your attention to your breathing. Can you feel it? Can you hear each breath and feel its journey into your lungs? Take a minute to adjust your breathing. Draw long, deep breaths in through your nose, to the count of four footsteps. Hold this breath in your chest for two steps, then gently release the air through pursed lips to the count of four footsteps. Repeat this rhythmic cycle, focusing on the journey of each breath.

- If your mind begins to wander, turn your attention back to the rhythmic footfall and your breathing. Try and keep this going for at least a few minutes, then pause and check in with yourself. How do you feel right now? Has the deep, steady breathing helped you feel calmer? If you are still feeling stressed, try this breathing cycle again for a couple of minutes.

- Once you have mastered this breathing technique, take things a step further. Imagine that with each breath you are drawing in the stillness of the water. Inhale this calming energy and visualize it traveling around your body in a wave of coolness. Look at the water as you do this; whether you're strolling by a river, lake, reservoir, or canal, focus on the serenity of the water and the way it flows gently. Listen to the sound made by the water, the relaxing lull as it rolls onward. Let this inspire you as you walk. Feel the water enveloping your body, giving you the flexibility to move freely. As you exhale, imagine the water pouring from you in one long breath. Continue to breathe in this way for the rest of your walk.

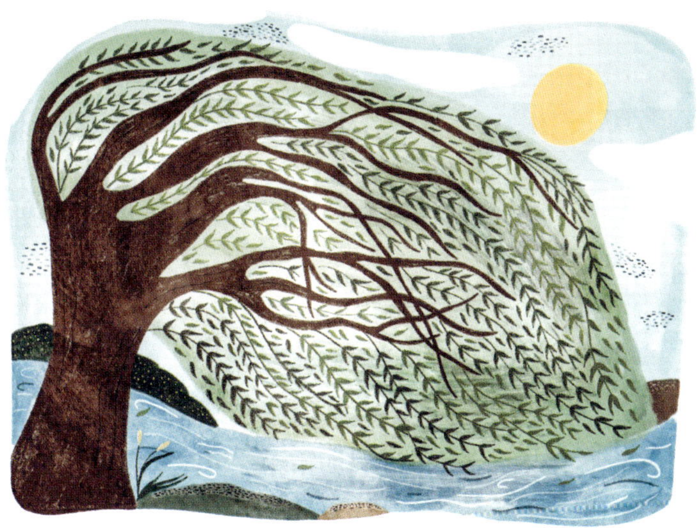

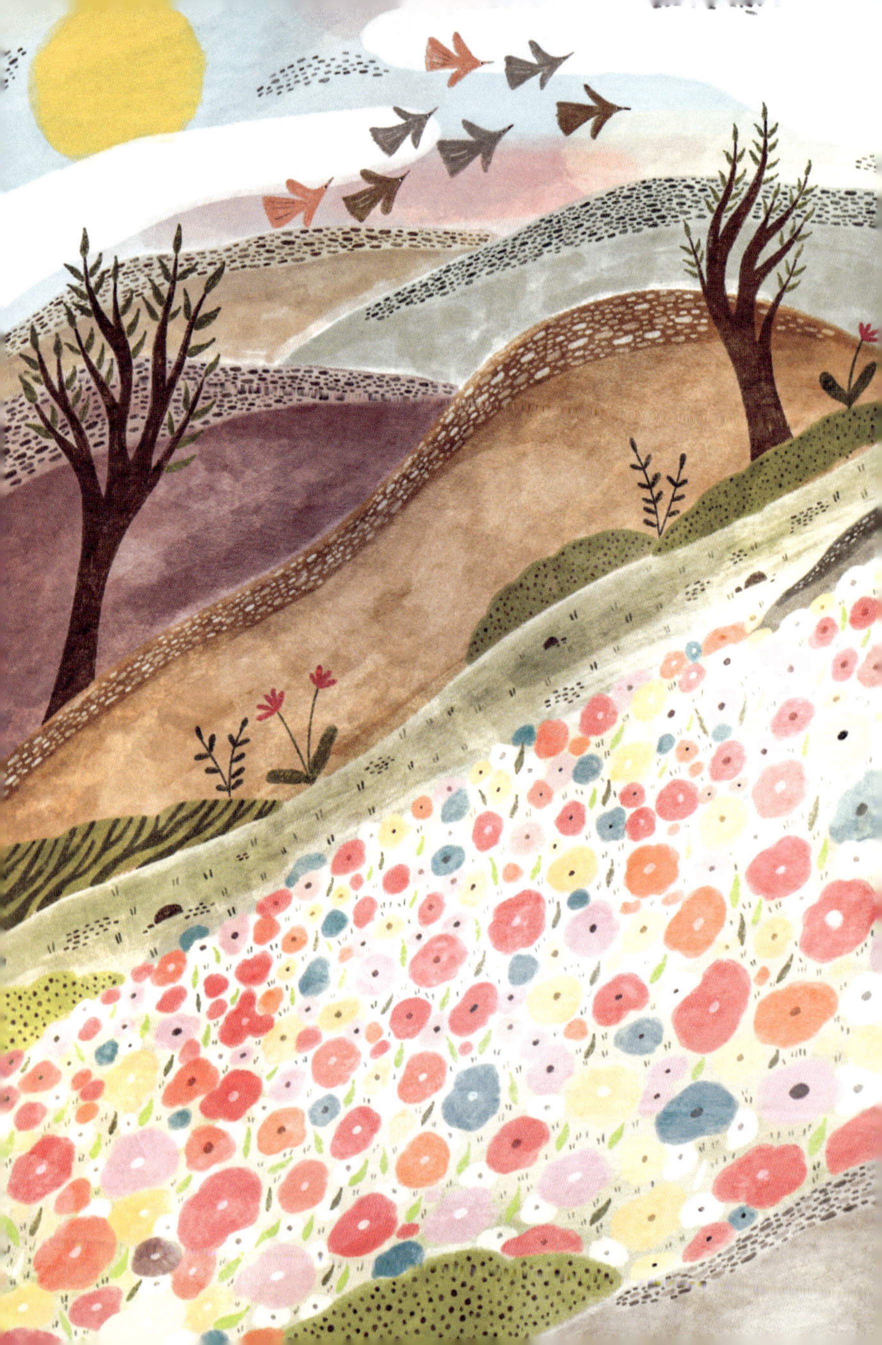

CHAPTER SIX

Mountains AND Meadows

Once you have mastered a short walk or a countryside amble, you might fancy something longer and more strenuous. The walks in this chapter are meant to challenge the body and mind, while also providing you with a well-being boost.

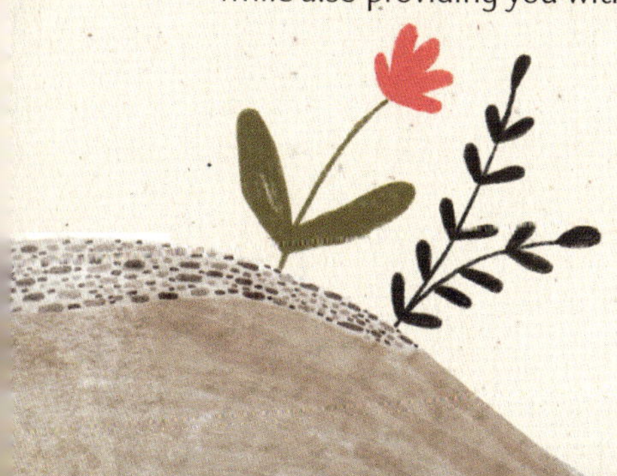

Strive for the Summit

Climbing any kind of slope is a challenge: whether you choose a mound, a hill, or a mountain, you'll need to take your time and put the effort in. The physical activity involved tests each muscle group, but it's particularly tough on the back, legs, and stomach. Arms and shoulders will also feel the weight of this workout.

If you can incorporate a slope into a longer hike, you'll improve your general body strength, stamina, and overall resilience. Your mental agility will also receive a boost, as you focus on each step.

CELEBRATE YOUR ACHIEVEMENTS

Reaching the top is exhilarating because you have achieved your goal. You set an intention with a target in mind, took the right steps to get there, and you made it! Mark this victory in some way. For instance, you might sit down and treat yourself to a snack, take some pictures of the glorious view, or find a memento of your journey, like an interesting stone or pretty pebble that you find at the summit. However you celebrate, seal the deal by making a positive statement such as, "I reached my goal. I carry this victory into everything I do!" Use this affirmation when you need a confidence boost, and it will remind you of the feeling you experienced at the end of your walk.

HILL HIKE

When you're walking up a slope, particularly over hilly terrain, you need to keep your wits about you. The concentration involved gives the mind a much-needed break from everyday concerns. Instead, put your focus on the environment and learn to read the landscape with every step you take.

Whether you're a solo walker or part of a group, nature is your guide, aiding your progress by providing a stimulating vista that you can use to propel yourself forward. With this in mind, it's a great time to take stock of where you are going in life, and what you hope to achieve. Use the challenge of the walk to fire up your aspirations for the future!

- Be prepared. Consider the weather and the terrain that you'll be walking over in advance. Wear appropriate clothing and walking boots with a good support; take a backpack stocked with energy-boosting snacks, water, and a first aid kit. Other helpful items to include are a flashlight, a fully charged phone, and spare clothing. It's also a good idea, if you're going to be on your own, to let somewhere know where you're headed.

- Take your time. This is a longer hike, so there's no need to rush. Use your senses to fully appreciate every step. Take in the panoramic views and notice the changes in the landscape as you climb. What kind of plants and trees can you see? How does the outlook change as you get higher? Take in the shifting hues and textures, the feel of the ground underfoot, and the scent of the air. Feel the shift in temperature and notice the breeze upon your face. Let this sensual experience push you onward.

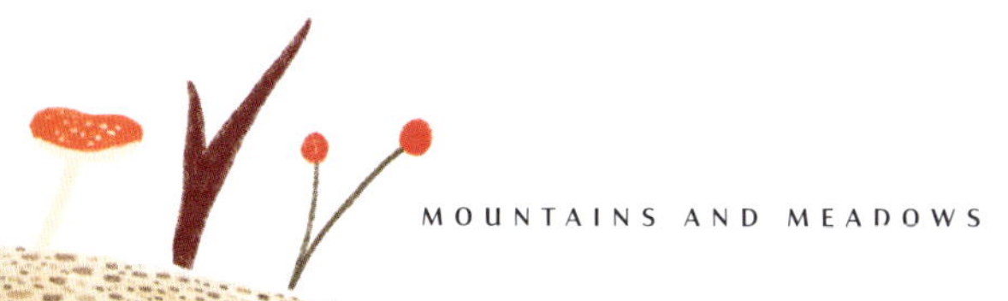

- Breathe deeply. Imagine you're drawing breath from the earth up into your lungs. Breathe through your nose and exhale slowly through your mouth. If you need to stop to take a breath, do so. Pause, inhale, and relax. Use this moment of stillness to reflect upon your progress so far. Look how far you have come and acknowledge this achievement.

- When you reach the top, take a moment to reflect. Appreciate the journey that you have taken, the highs and lows, and how difficult it was. Acknowledge the effort that you have put in. Drink in the bird's-eye view—how the landscape unfolds before you. Consider other goals in your life—these could be work-related or personal—and the steps you have taken so far to attain them. Know that you are resilient and have the strength to achieve anything you set your mind to—as this walk has just proved!

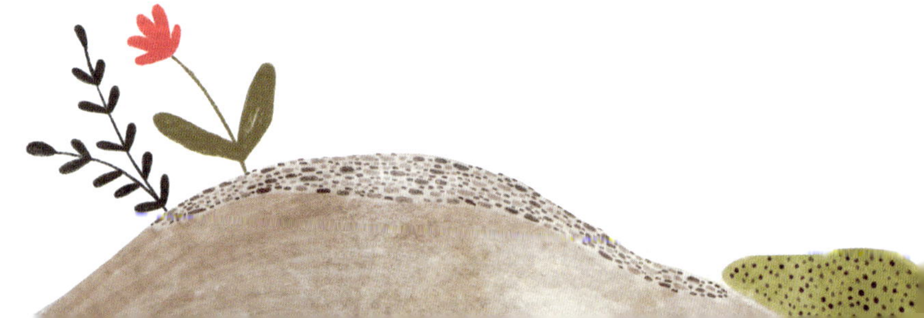

WALK 47

Run Through the Meadow

Each landscape has something different to offer; a feast for the eyes that varies depending on the season and the time of day. A meadow ramble in the spring has a different feel to a long walk through the fields on a hot summer's day, when the blades of grass burn golden under the midday sun. An autumn amble offers a vibrant color palette that makes you feel warm on the coldest day, while winter has its own charm tinged with icy clarity and wide, open spaces.

If you want to observe the changes, choose a stretch of meadow for a long walk through the seasons, starting with some spring fun!

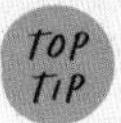

LOG YOUR FINDS

Document your finds by taking pictures on your phone. This is particularly effective when it comes to wildflowers and herbs, as you'll then be able to recognize them again. If you prefer, keep a notebook and write a short description to help you identify each plant. Logging your finds in this way helps to cement memories of your walks.

SPRING MEADOW SPOTTING

Turn a spring meadow foray into a game. You can do this on your own or with family and friends. Either way, you'll hone your observation skills and have lots of fun interacting with nature.

- Before you set off, make a list of all things you're likely to see on your ramble. Consider the different types of wildlife: As the warmer season returns, fields and meadows are a great place to spot butterflies like the small white, burnet moths, grasshoppers, various types of beetles, and bees. If you're patient you might see voles and mice, or frogs and toads if the field is near water, and rabbits or hares (if you are lucky) grazing in the tall grasses. Ground-nesting birds like skylarks, curlews, and meadow pipits can be spotted with a keen eye. Also look out for birds of prey like kestrels and buzzards as they might be hunting in the area.

- Notice the time of day that you are taking the walk, as this will affect what you see. For example, if you go out later in the evening, you might see owls hunting, bats in search of a tasty morsel, and a variety of moths or fireflies.

- If you have a favorite meadow walk, you can vary your spotting theme, so you might want to stick to wildflowers and herbs one day, and focus solely on birds or insects another.

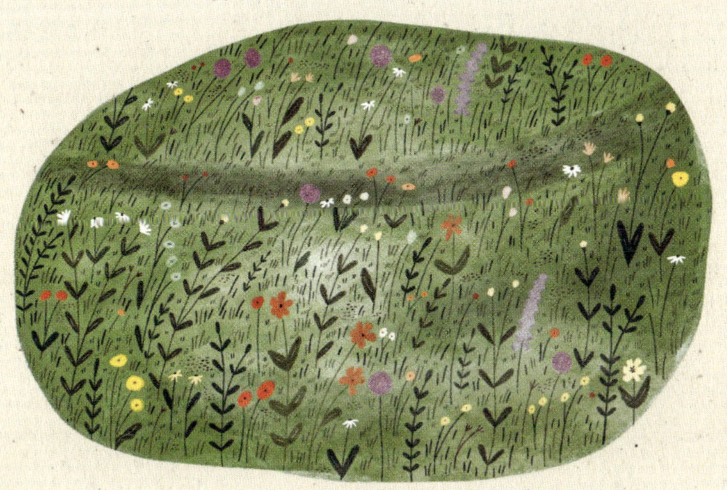

THINGS TO LOOK OUT FOR:

To get you started, here's a list of common wildflowers that you might spot while on out on your walk:

Oxeye Daisy
Common in grassy fields and meadows, this bloom has a halo of white petals and a yellow center.

Cowslip
Nodding yellow blooms, which usually appear in spring and favor meadows and forests.

Meadow Buttercup These tall, bright buttercups are often found in hay meadows.

Red and White Clover
Usually found in abundance in pastures and meadows.

Also look out for: Field poppies in a range of hues, cornflowers, black knapweed, and red campion.

WALK 48

Listen and Learn

Evidence suggests that exposure to birds in any form is beneficial for those suffering with depression. The melodic pattern of birdsong is similar to the gentle rhythm of a lullaby, and known to induce a sense of calm, while the sounds of nature in general are thought to lower the heart rate and promote feel-good neurotransmitters like dopamine and serotonin. Researchers have discovered that natural noise regulates the body's autonomic nervous system, taking it from "fight or flight" to "rest and digest."

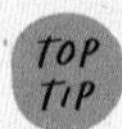

LET THE SOUNDS GUIDE YOU

Don't be afraid to divert from the path if you hear an interesting noise. This walk is about stimulating the senses and engaging with the natural world, so if something piques your interest, go with it. Follow the strand of sound and see if you can identify where it is coming from. Be alert and let nature reveal itself to you note by note.

HEALING SOUND RAMBLE

A longer hike is the perfect opportunity to reconnect with the natural world. If you walk with the intention of listening, you'll be pleasantly surprised by the many layers of sound that greet your ears. From twittering songbirds to the calming rustle of the wind through the trees, the symphony of nature is at its most potent when the landscape is mixed, so seek out a ramble that takes you through meadows, heathland, and riversides, and you'll benefit from a range of healing sounds.

STEP 1 *Step gently, so you can tune into the landscape.* At first, you'll notice surface sounds, the noise of your own feet as they crunch along the path or squelch through mud and grass, the murmuring chatter of other walkers, or dogs barking in the distance. Acknowledge this first layer of sound, pinpoint each thread, and where it is coming from, then let it go.

STEP 2 *Breathe deeply and let each inhalation soothe you.* This walk should be relaxing. The calmer you feel, the more likely you are to pick up different levels of sound. Scan your surroundings for clues, so you might look high in the sky and notice a couple of birds of prey circling—pause and see if you can hear their distinctive call. You might see a group of gulls flying overhead and hear their throaty cries. Gaze into the hedgerows and seek out movement. You might hear the rustle of a tiny bird like a wren, or spot a squirrel darting through the undergrowth. Your eyes are the partner to your ears, and they will direct you to new and interesting noises.

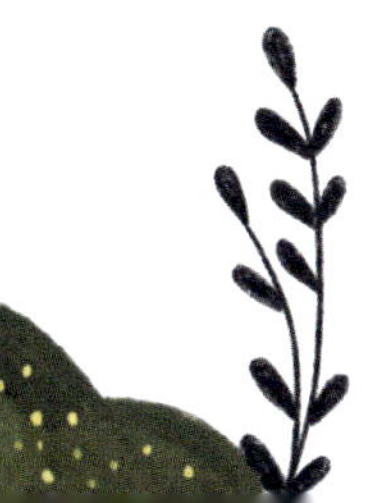

STEP 3 ***Walk on and settle into the musical cadence of nature.*** Notice how there are many layers of sound beneath the surface. Identify each one and where it sits in the great symphony. For example, the rushing wind that surges through the trees provides the base note, a low, whooshing hum of background noise that calms the mind. Then there are the higher notes—the fluting sounds of birdsong from one side, a different kind of chirruping coming from the other. Consider what type of bird might be making each noise and where this sits in the musical overture. From the river you might hear a warbling or a squawking cry from a pair of ducks, the noise of a wader as it takes flight, or the sound of one landing clumsily in the reeds. Identify each thread of sound and follow it to its source.

STEP 4 ***Let your focus fade from each distinctive note and allow your mind and senses to rest.*** Take a moment to let the entire orchestra play, and enjoy the sounds of nature as a whole. Consider where you fit into this. What sound do you add? Perhaps you are simply keeping pace as you walk, adding a slow, steady rhythm to this piece of music. Enjoy the rest of your walk by staying present and listening to the many levels of sound that envelop you.

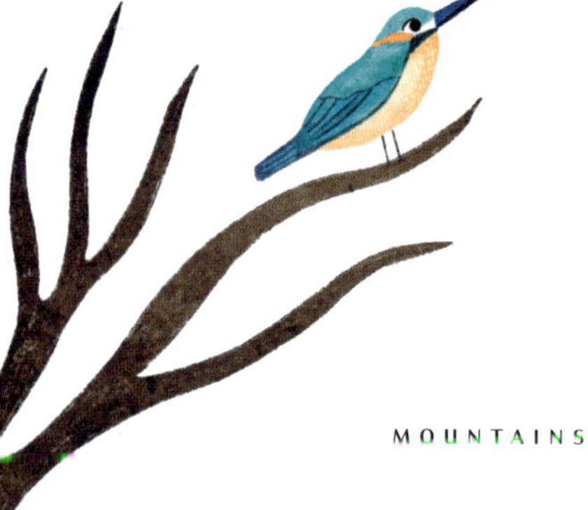

WALK 49

Conquer New Ground

Hiking is healthy. It strengthens the body and mind, exercises joints and muscles, and reduces the risk of heart disease, dementia, and some cancers. A brisk walk makes the heart work harder, pumping blood and oxygen around your body, which over time strengthens the muscles of the heart and improves their function.

Each step on uneven terrain works the muscles and acts like a weight-bearing workout. The stress that this places, particularly on the bones in the legs and lower back, strengthens and stimulates bone-forming cells, which improves overall bone density. Couple this effect with the lengthy exposure to sunlight that boosts vitamin D, a key vitamin in bone health, and you have a natural remedy for brittle bones.

Longer hikes offer the opportunity to break new ground and vary your walking pace. Changing up the speed and effort challenges the body and mind and keeps things exciting.

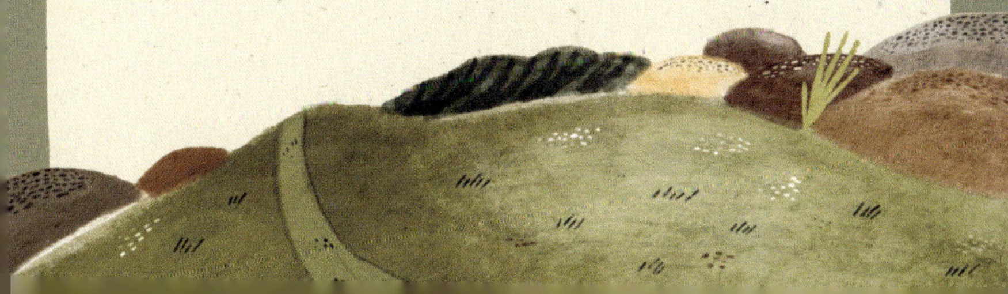

HEART-HEALTHY RAMBLE

Engage body and mind in a long and varied walk, which challenges you in different ways. Choose a shifting environment and match this with the speed and length of your stride to help you navigate the changes.

- Be prepared. This type of hike will take you over mixed terrain, so wear good, solid boots with lots of ankle support. You might want to invest in some walking poles to help you navigate the landscape and support your knees. Also, carry plenty of water with you and some energy snacks in a backpack.

- Work with the environment. Adjust your gait to suit the landscape, so if you're walking uphill, take longer, slower strides to help you balance and cover the ground. Breathe deeply to fuel each step. If you're walking on a flat section, take shorter steps and pick up speed. Inhale in short, sharp bursts and exhale deeply.

- Think about each step you take and what you need to do to keep going. Be aware of your surroundings and stay focused.

- Vary your speed. The landscape may dictate your pace, but if it's fairly steady all the way you can vary it yourself by having periods of brisk walking.

- Set a timer and start small, especially if you're not an experienced walker. Set your alarm for ten minutes. During this time, you're going to pick up the pace, breathe deeply, and get your heart rate up. Once the time is up, return to a steady pace for five minutes.

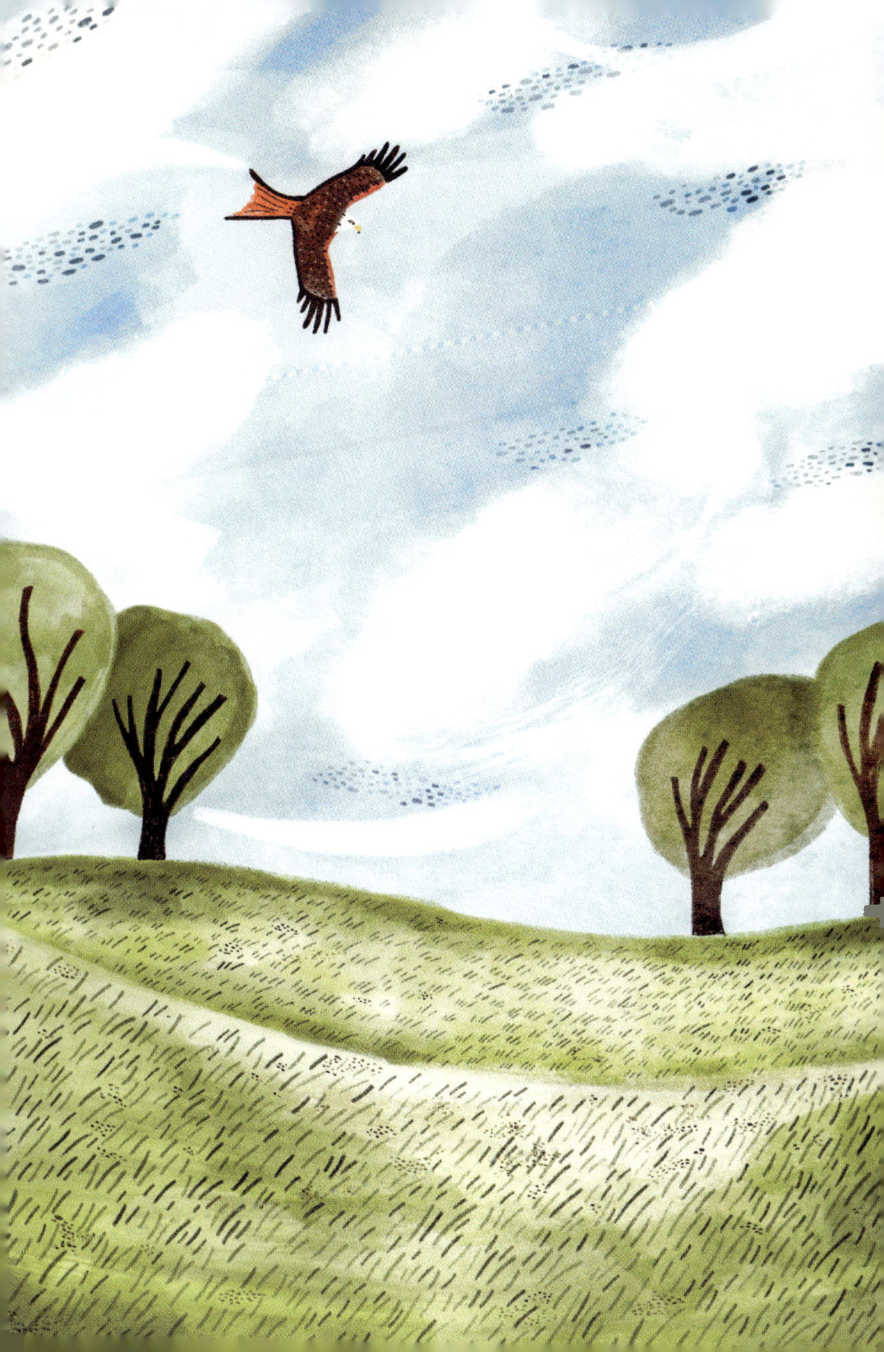

- Build up to longer periods of brisk walking, so you might set the timer for twenty minutes the next time.

- Stick to a maximum of thirty minutes brisk walking, then return to a normal pace and give yourself a breather.

- If you need a break, stop. Pause and take in the view. Allow yourself breathing space. Your aim is to exercise and strengthen the heart, but to feel the benefits fully you need to have short resting periods.

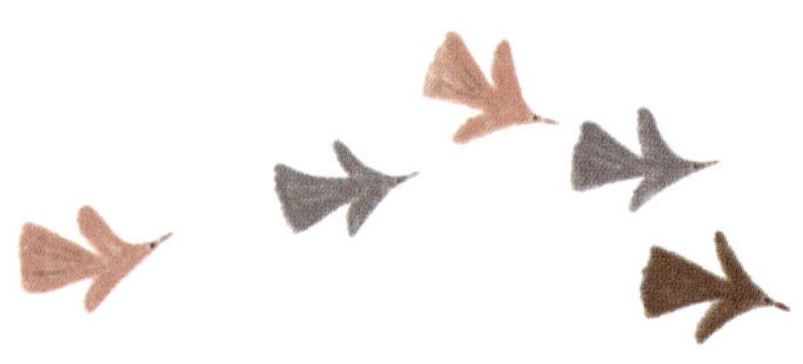

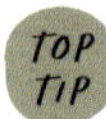

TAKE TIME TO STRETCH OUT

Perform a few simple stretches during your rest period. This will soothe tired muscles and keep you flexible during your hike. A forward lunge, where you bend one knee forward and the other leg back, either straight or slightly bent, helps to keep the hips flexible. To stretch out hamstrings, place one leg on a higher surface like a stone step or large boulder and stretch forward gently from the hips; you should feel the pull in your thigh or knee. Don't forget your arms and shoulders. Shake them out and do a few shoulder rolls, lifting them up to your ears and then rolling them back and down; repeat this circular motion five to ten times in each direction.

WALK 50

Read and Reap Rewards

Meadows and mountains are the perfect canvas to ponder. With an array of sights and sounds and no need to rush, you can truly engage as you walk. Sense the way forward and take inspiration from the rise and fall of the earth beneath your feet. If you're feeling weary, simply take each step slowly and let the landscape guide you in a natural meditation.

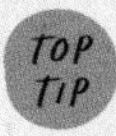

DON'T FORGET TO REST

Rest at regular intervals. Like any form of exercise, you'll need to take breaks. This is a longer walk and the intention is to reduce stress rather than put pressure on yourself. Each time the environment changes, give yourself a moment to adjust. Take in the shifting views, and have some water and a snack if you feel you need it, to replenish yourself physically. Take a couple of energizing breaths and stretch out sore limbs before you begin the next phase. Your body and mind will thank you.

MINDFUL MEDITATION TREK

As well as benefiting your bones, a long ramble gives you the time and space to breathe and disengage from the busy world of ten thousand things. When you pay attention to the fluctuating landscape, to the rise and fall of the earth beneath your feet, it soothes the brain and provides the downtime you need to ponder deeper issues. Even if you want to completely switch off and recharge, you'll find what you need with some mindful meditation as you ramble.

STEP 1 *To begin, have a route in mind and familiarize yourself with it on a map.* Make sure you have everything you need to navigate your way safely. If possible, choose a route that takes you through different settings. For example, you could begin walking through a field that leads to an uphill hike, which then takes you down by a stream into a meadow.

STEP 2 *This walk is about alleviating stress, so take your time and relax.* Loosen your shoulders and arms by shaking them out. Take comfortable strides and place your attention on each footfall, and how the ground feels beneath your boots.

STEP 3 *Breathe deeply and with purpose.* Imagine that with each breath you're drawing in an element of your surroundings. For example, you might drink in the lushness of the green field at your feet, the fresh blades of grass with their sweet scent that you can taste upon the tip of your tongue. Perhaps it's the fusion of vibrant wildflowers that catches your eye, so draw in a breath that captures the essence of this floral carpet. Maybe it's the sky that draws your interest, and so you inhale this vast sea of softness and feel the cooling energy soothe your mind.

STEP 4 *As you walk, find different things to appreciate,* features that embody the beauty of nature and fill you with wonder, like the cluster of trees that look almost human as they weave in the breeze, or the sun dancing upon the rolling fields, making them shine like a golden sea.

STEP 5 *Notice the rhythm of your gait and how it changes,* depending on where you are. For example, if you're climbing a slope, you might take longer, slower steps, while a smooth plateau of land is easier to navigate, so you pick up speed and let your arms swing in time with each step.

STEP 6 *Feel your way forward, taking the lead from the landscape around you.* Be aware of where you are, and where you are going, and let this be the focus of your thoughts. Know that in life too, you can take your time and just go with the flow, rather than charging on and forcing a path.

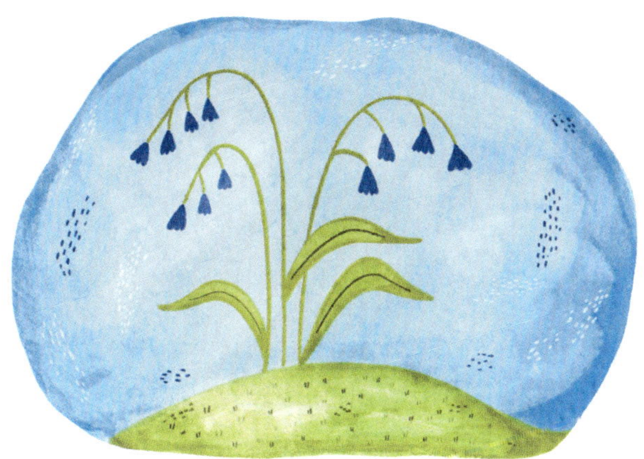

Index

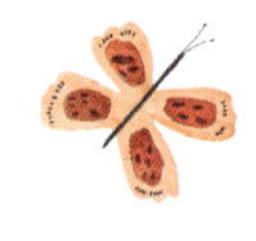

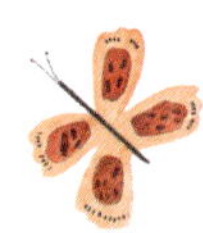

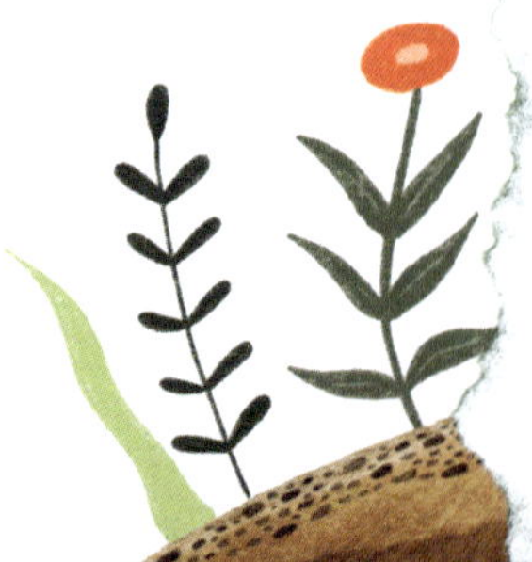